STAY FIT STAY LIT

A COMPLETE GUIDE TO HOLISTIC WELLNESS

SAMUDRA B

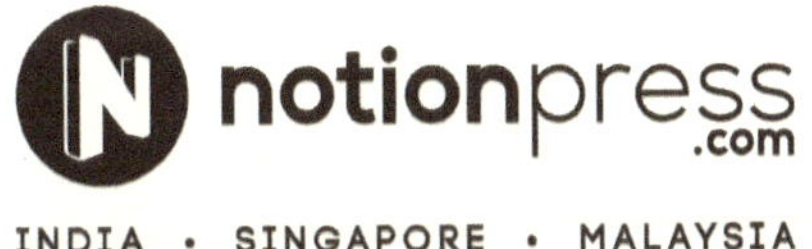

Contents

Introduction

My mum always says, "Wealth is nothing without your health. Creating wealth means different things to different people, but for me, besides making money, wealth means that you're fit, strong, and healthy and that you're wealthy in terms of your relationships with your family and friends and in every other aspect of your life."

The healthier you are, the longer you can enjoy the fruits of your labour. Your body is like a vehicle; caring for it ensures optimal performance.

It's important to prioritise how you look after yourself, how you treat your body, what you eat, and alter your bad habits. This book is for anyone who is looking for motivation, wants to feel active and energised. Even on the days when you have nothing much to do, you must feel good about yourself.

Why should people exercise?

Exercise is a natural stress buster. Spending some time in enjoyable physical activity changes your focus and is a well-deserved break from your regular routine.

People at work find it very hard to take a break from their routines. I was recently at Passport Seva Kendra for a mental wellness programme as a speaker to address the audience about health. I met and interacted with a group of young people who expressed their lack of motivation and consistency towards health. The truth is not many people are simply motivated enough to begin an exercise routine. It was disheartening to see the youngsters not being so consciously aware about health.

You may view exercise as something that is too boring, too much work, or something that is just not for you.

Many people start exercise plans over and over again only to quit. For some people, they don't see changes in the body fast enough and become discouraged. For others, they are just not having fun.

- Do you want to feel motivated?

- Do you want to feel energised?

- Do you want to thrive at work?

- Do you want to be the best in whatever you do?

Then this book is certainly for you, and you have made the right choice. This book will help you ignite that joie de vivre.

Chapter 1

You Are the Sum of Your Habits

We become what we repeatedly do - Stephen Covey

The first step towards forming a habit is awareness,

So, who are you? What are the habits that define you?

If you want to be a writer?, you must practise writing every day.

If you want to finish a triathlon? You will need to train daily.

If you want to be an artist?, you need to paint every day. Think about the activities you perform regularly. My suggestion is to start slow. One habit at a time. Your unrealised habits are more ingrained than you can imagine.

For example: look for something that isn't good for your health, then show your brain that you have the discipline to make decisions for yourself rather than letting outside forces control you.

List small actionable changes you can incorporate daily for progress.

These can be very small changes. Instead of having bread or a bun for breakfast, be conscious enough to consume good portions of fruits; have a banana instead. Try to think of 5 small changes you can make that could add another 5 or 10 years to your life.

If you are honest in your approach, you will notice many things holding you back from growth. Changing will take massive effort, which eventually leads to ease. That is what makes habits amazing.

We often believe that major transformations in life come from huge dramatic shifts - a sudden change in direction, a life-altering decision or an overwhelming burst of motivation. But what if I told you it's not the big changes but the small, consistent actions that truly drive lasting success? Small wins are those tiny incremental steps that may feel insignificant at the start, but over time, they compound into monumental progress. It's about the daily, seemingly insignificant choices that, compounded over time, lead to massive results.

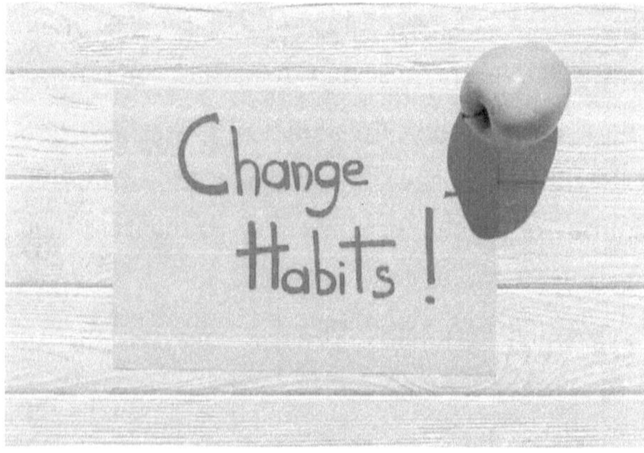

My mornings always consist of the following activities:

1. Surya Namaskar (sun salutations)

2. Pranayama

3. Affirmations

4. Meditation

5. Gratitude

6. Deep breathing

Let's examine it from the reverse perspective.

Are you overweight?

Out of shape? Underachieving? Lost? As society increases in complexity, younger generations struggle to define themselves. When you focus on building a habit, you orient yourself to a much healthier game.

Living life from my perspective:

Life changes for everybody. Coronavirus has made me want to fast forward my plans. I've had all the rush and pressure of our society.

There is a constant need to achieve or prove yourself.

The unspoken message is that if you are not being productive or showing your worth by doing something, then you are being lazy or a slacker.

I've never bought into the regular 9 am-6 pm kind of life, the pursuit of more, working my way up the career ladder. Even when I was at university, nothing in me was attracted to the graduate training programme with top companies. My mother, being my biggest support system, always believed in my freedom and autonomy. I quit the rat race and was more than contended to go towards my inner calling to lead a simple life. Through meditation, I have constantly sought answers to all the critical decisions of my life. I have defined my own version of success in life.

For me, true success in life is measured by the degree of peace, joy, and love we experience and share.

Life has given me many opportunities to learn, become better and inculcate some good habits. To a great extent, when I say, 'life has given me many opportunities', it's the background and support I got from my mother and a few loving friends. After pandemic, our business took a bad shape and we hit a very uncertain low phase in life. When you have a close encounter with highs and lows, when you are just hanging by a thread and don't have any idea what will happen the very next moment, you start working hard, utilising each second that you have, valuing the people around you, and observing the world from a totally different perspective.

In essence, if we want to direct our lives, we must take control of our consistent actions. It's not what we do once in a while that shapes our lives, but what we do consistently. – Tony Robbins

I have made it a conscious choice to keep my mornings productive. Unproductive mornings lead to a lack of self-discipline or drive. Getting up in the morning and getting distracted by emails or social media is something that we have all done at some point in life. In general, I have a positive mindset, but it is something that I have been cultivating for many years now; practising gratitude is one of the more significant habits I have instilled in recent years. I say thank you first thing in the morning and last thing at night; I say thank you for specific things in my life. Gratitude has worked like a magic pill.

From my personal experience,

I have been practising gratitude for a decade now. Through gratitude, I have experienced paradigm shifts taking place in my life. I have gone through many ups and downs, but when I moved into the space of gratitude, these seeming losses – which were actually gifts - enabled me to be in the flow of life.

One of the best ways to practise mindfulness and gratitude is to start and end your day with a clear and positive intention, which is what I normally do.

Exercise:

Start your day

Before you get out of bed, take a few moments to breathe deeply.

INHALE AND EXHALE.

- Slowly bring your focus to the surroundings

- Notice how your body feels

- What sounds do you hear?

- What emotions do you feel? A positive mindset can bring you to a state of thankfulness

- Then, set an intention for your day, such as being kind, productive, or creative

- You can also express gratitude for something or someone in your life, such as Health, family, friends, and opportunities

Ending Your Day

End your day with reflection. Before you go to sleep, take some time to reflect on your day and acknowledge your learnings, achievements, and challenges.

You can also list a few things you are grateful for in a journal. This will help you recognise the good in your life.

You can also meditate, pray, relax, & do some mild breathing exercises before retiring to bed.

This will help you to sleep better, reduce stress, and enhance your overall well-being.

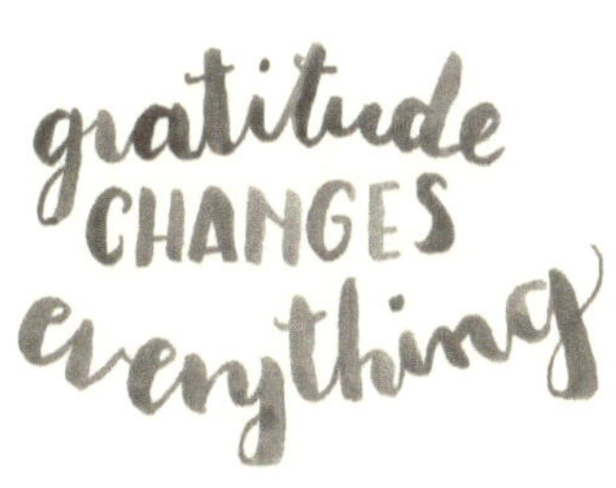

At times, before going to bed, I say these affirmations out loud:

- I am grateful for my body

- I am grateful for this day

- I am grateful to be alive

- Gratitude fills my heart with joy

- The universe is supporting me and working in my favour

- I exhale worry and inhale gratitude

- Good things are coming my way

- I am surrounded by healing energy

- I am open to all kinds of blessings and miracles

- I am grateful for my friends and family

Gratitude Exercise while eating:

- Choose one of the foods you're eating

- Imagine the journey it took to get to your plate

All the people who worked to get it there. (Someone planted it, fertilised it, and transported it) We owe all those people behind the scenes huge thanks.

Gratitude Is A Game-changer:

Life won't necessarily go your way forever. If adversity strikes, it can be difficult to recall a time when you were grateful. Our days are filled with moments, both big and small, that shape our lives. Sometimes, in the hustle of daily responsibilities, we forget to pause and reflect on these moments. Gratitude is the ultimate biohack. It reduces stress, improves sleep, and strengthens your immune system. A grateful heart is essential for health. There are so many good things that you can think about while journaling. You can think of something as simple as:

- **Writing about a time when you laughed uncontrollably**

- **Appreciating a friend who lives far away but is dear to you**

- **A movie that touched your heart**, Gratitude journaling is writing about anything that reminds you of life's magic. Knowing, loving, and being grateful for yourself all start by exploring the inner you - your inward swirl of emotions, energies, and abilities. Write everything you can remember to figure out what has brought you joy recently and what you can do to keep chasing that feeling. A few years ago, I started writing in a gratitude journal that someone gave me as a gift. In the beginning, I simply tried to write 7 things each morning for which I was grateful. The practice encouraged me to look back on the past 24 hours and recall all the good aspects of the day. Through this simple practice, I also discovered I was more aware of special moments and simple blessings that occurred in my life. I soon started filling the little book and began another. To my joy of discovery, I made it a practice, and today, it's my quiet way of reflecting in the mornings. I have now realised that it is my calling and passion to share the power of gratitude to inspire others.

If you are wondering how and where to start, here are some prompts you could write about in your gratitude journal.

- **A supportive friend or family member who has constantly been there for you**

- **A memorable experience or event that brought you joy or happiness**

- **Time spent with your pet if you have one**

- **The beauty of nature, such as a stunning sunrise, sunset, or a blooming flower**

- **A delicious meal with friends or a favourite outing that brought you comfort or pleasure**

- **A favourite book, movie, or piece of art that has inspired or influenced you**

To be able to experience gratitude, you don't need any grand gestures. Gratitude can be found in the simplest things. There are more simple things to focus on when it comes to gratitude:

- Life - for giving you the chance to experience all that you are experiencing and will be experiencing in time to come

- Life's challenges - for letting you grow and become who you are

- Laughter and all the lighter moments - for connecting you to closer to fulfilling and a more meaningful relationships

- Your best friends - for being there for you whenever you need them

- Your home - a place you can call home

- Music - for lifting your spirits when you feel life has doomed you or filling life with more love

- Your job - to provide you with a source of living

- Technology - for making all the impossible things possible

- Books - for adding wisdom to life. The time spent reading is most resourceful

- Mobile - for keeping you connected with the ever-growing and evolving world

- Happy moments - to soak in all the beauty of life

- Parents - for giving birth

- Family - for being the closest kin in the world

- Speech - for giving you the outlet to express yourself

- Lungs - for letting you breathe and experience the miraculous joy of staying alive

- Eyes - that give you the vision to see the world

- Ears - to hear the music and laughter

- Nose – to smell flowers, freshly baked cookies, and perfumes that linger in the air

- Tongue – to taste all your favourite foods

- Resilient, self-repairing skin that shields and protects you from all harsh environmental conditions

- The immune system is used to fight against the viruses that enter your body. For keeping you in the pink of health so you can do the things you love doing

- Sadness and pain help you become a stronger person, helping you appreciate the spectrum of human emotions

The list I have shared above is very basic; there are millions of things to be grateful for. You will find them once you dig a little deeper into your life. Millions are still deprived of necessities for survival. People fight a constant battle each day to make ends meet and are deprived of life. One of the prime reasons behind people's constant discontent with life is not appreciating what you already possess. So, never spare a chance to be grateful.

Studies have found that focusing on the positive things in life can help reduce stress, improve sleep, and even be good for our personal relationships. I get stressed when I'm feeling critical and focused on the things that aren't happening according to my expectations. What I have noticed is that when I make a deliberate effort to see my life through the eyes of a grateful heart, I am more accepting of my situation and content.

Chapter 2

Raising Health Concerns

India, being the most populated country in the world, also has the highest number of patients suffering from chronic health issues.

The following are the factors that are contributing to health issues in the younger population.

- Consumption of processed foods
- Sedentary lifestyle
- Excessive use of tobacco and alcohol
- Chronic stress
- Pollution
- Expensive medical care

Obesity:

Obesity has become an epidemic in India. Young kids, as well as adults, are equally struggling with physical issues like BMI, body fat, etc.

Reduced outdoor playtime, fattening junk food, and sitting all day in the comfort of AC have made kids more prone to obesity.

Cardio Vascular:

Cardiovascular diseases are among the most common health problems and the top factor causing death among younger and older populations. Blockage in arteries is the most common health issue. Most heart conditions can be altered and are preventable with a change in diet and lifestyle.

Cancer:

It is the second most common disease in India among the younger and older population. The most common forms of cancer in India are oral, breast, lung, stomach, and cervical. This can be treated at an early stage and can also be prevented by maintaining a healthy and balanced lifestyle.

Chronic Respiratory Disease:

High air pollution, smoking, use of biomass fuel, and poor living conditions are major factors contributing to a rise in respiratory diseases such as chronic obstructive pulmonary disease and bronchitis.

The breathing techniques to maintain a healthy lifestyle are highlighted in the later chapters of this book. Practising those techniques will reduce asthma and bronchial conditions.

Diabetes:

India is known to have the highest cases of diabetes in the world. It is characterised by high blood sugar levels. It is the biggest health threat in India today. Diabetes is a major health concern among children as young as 12 years old due to poor lifestyles and unhealthy habits.

Hypertension:

High blood pressure is one of the most common health concerns. It is the leading factor causing a stroke and a heart attack. It is caused by physical inactivity, stress, and unhealthy habits.

Chronic Kidney Disease:

Chronic kidney disease is caused by many other underlying medical issues, such as obesity, hypertension, diabetes, etc. It is a slow-progressing disease causing failure over time.

Reason: dietary and lifestyle changes.

Reproductive Health Issues:

Reproductive health issues, particularly one in 5 women suffer from reproductive issues. Changing lifestyles and pressure to maintain a work-life balance (the dual responsibility of career and household work) have led to a rise in cases of PCOD and infertility.

Mental Health Issues:

Lately, the cases of mental health disorders such as depression, anxiety, OCD, bipolar disorder, and substance abuse have increased. Bringing awareness and integration with primary health care can help reduce stigma.

Depression and anxiety are among the leading causes of illness and disability among adolescents.

So, for all the above-discussed health issues, powerful medicine exists. It's real and readily available for everyone.

It is called the 'intensive lifestyle change'.

Its active ingredients are:

- Physical activity

- Drastic improvement in diet

- Good sleep

If it were an actual pill, millions of people would be clamouring for it and some pharmaceutical company would be reaping massive profits.

Intensive lifestyle change involves knowledge + action.

Bad behaviours such as drinking, smoking, and overeating are actually people's attempts to self-medicate emotional pain. Distracting your mind with good habits can be a helpful way to divert your attention from addictions.

The power of exercise alone can put an end to all our health-related concerns. Did you know that the power of exercising for just 30 minutes a day can lower the risk of developing 13 types of cancer? They aren't just any cancers; they are primarily metabolic cancers that directly respond to lifestyle changes.

Research reveals that people who start exercising after a cancer diagnosis have significantly higher survival rates, especially those diagnosed with breast, prostate, and colon cancers. So make exercise a daily habit; it's one of the most powerful tools you have for preventing and fighting against cancer.

Incorporating movement not only enhances physical health but also nurtures mental clarity, bringing balance to your life. A combination of healthy lifestyle choices such as maintaining a healthy weight, not smoking, and regularly exercising can significantly extend the number of years an individual avoids disease.

Altering your lifestyle factors can make a significant difference in the risk of disease and length of life overall. A healthful lifestyle not only decreases the risk of cardiovascular disease, type 2 diabetes, and cancer but also improves survival after the diagnosis of those diseases.

Chapter 3

Move Your Body

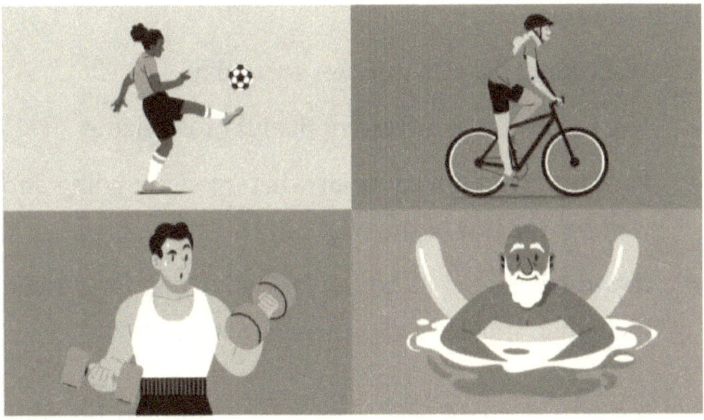

Living a sedentary lifestyle can be dangerous to your health. The less time you spend sitting or lying down during the day, the better your chances of leading a healthy lifestyle.

Humans are built to stand upright. Your heart and cardiovascular system work more effectively. Your bowel also functions more efficiently when you are upright. Sitting for long hours can lead to varicose veins or spider veins. This is because long hours of sitting cause blood to pool in your legs.

Long hours of sitting can stiffen your neck, shoulders, and joints. If you spend time hunched over a laptop, TV, or work desk for long hours, it will lead to pain and stiffness in your neck and shoulders.

For every half an hour of sitting, take a stroll or move around for a few minutes. Building more activity into your day is important.

Some ways you can incorporate activity into your daily life are:

- Walk for at least 30 minutes every day

- Use the staircase instead of the lift or escalator

- Parking further away from where you are going and walking the rest of the way

- If you have a pet at home, take your dog for a walk. (Schedule smaller walks throughout the day).

Hitting a step count goal day in and out can be quite monotonous. If you want to increase your step count, you must look for more enjoyable ways of doing it. Continue to use mindful awareness as you move your body. No matter the activity, the key is finding small, manageable ways to incorporate movement into your day.

Frequently acknowledging the state of your body is important:

- How does your body feel?

- Are you reaching your goal?

- Are you reaping the benefits?

Change your goal over time as needed.

When it comes to monitoring your wellness, consider writing a SMART goal.

- **Specific**: what exactly will you do?
- Answer: My target is to take a minimum of 5000 steps daily
- **Measurable**: How much and how often will you do it?
- Answer: I will incorporate at least weekly, 4 days into my routines
- **Action-oriented**: What action will you take?
- Answer: Walks for 30 minutes daily on my terrace, use stairs, move around to drink water frequently, take a break and stand upright, play with my pet, and do stretches
- **Realistic**: Is this a goal you can achieve?
- A: Yes, these goals are very much achievable and within my control
- **Timed**: when will you start and end?
- A: First hour of the morning every day (the first hours are meant for self-care and self-improvement) and anytime during the day and evenings

When you don't listen to your body's needs, you will end up feeling very disconnected. When you do listen to your body, you acknowledge it and you give it a voice. Nourishing your body with food when it's hungry, taking a few deep breaths when you find your body is tensing up are all ways to feel closer to your body. When you are unwell, giving the body required sleep and rest are all the ways you can repay your wonderful body.

Chapter 4

Lessons Learnt During Covid

The COVID-19 changed our lives as we know it.

From our morning routines to our life goals, everything got altered in those 2 years.

Very important lessons I reflected on through the pandemic were:

- **The Value of Life**: We are all given one life, and how we spend it depends on us

A few strong realisations dawned upon me within the first few months of lockdown.

- Life is not just about accumulating material things and achievements

- It is more than just being successful in terms of material riches

- Life is all about leaving behind a legacy of humility and love

The second most profound lesson I learnt was:

Simplifying your life not only reduces stress but also gives you more time to focus on health and relationships.

The world is filled with unnecessary complexities. The less you have, the more time you have to focus on the important things. Some things go beyond money, such as:

- **Valuing your health**
- **Quality time with your family and loved ones**
- **Practising gratitude**
- **Going the extra mile in helping others**
- **Valuing and prioritising yourself**

In the little time we have, let's be grateful for the people around us, be appreciative of the beauty that surrounds us, and be faithful to the God above us.

Covid-19 taught me the brevity of life. The pandemic gave me a better insight into health. Thriving in challenging times can be a herculean task. Stress is a normal response during a crisis, making it challenging to maintain a healthy lifestyle. But that's exactly when you need to maintain a healthy lifestyle.

We all have 24 hours at hand every day. We can get so much work done each day.

If we avoid procrastination and follow micro-goals, life will become hassle-free. Success lies in small daily habits. Hitting the gym is not the only way to maintain good health.

Being careless about seemingly small and simple things can deteriorate your health instead of helping you achieve your fitness goals.

During COVID-19, we saw a surge in online classes when the coronavirus forced schools and offices to shut their doors and move classes and work sessions online. Essentially, everyone was forced to become online learners.

Some wondered if traditional education would crumble as companies such as Google saw increased interest in online certificate programmes. In the last 2 years, the pandemic has propelled everyone to move forward greatly as entrepreneurs, businesses, and teachers pivoted online, resulting in a surge of new course creations.

The lockdown pushed the growth of online yoga classes.

"Yoga at home and yoga with family came into conceptualisation."

Due to the lockdown in place, many were stuck at home with very little to do. Because of the extra time, people became more interested and conscious about their health.

When the health and fitness centres were not functioning as usual, people were missing out on their daily dose of exercise.

That led many to look out for options like yoga, dance, and bodyweight workouts from the comfort of their home. Many fitness enthusiasts were happy that they were able to effectively work out even within the confines of their homes.

During these unprecedented times, I looked at making some micro changes. According to the World Health Organization, since the outbreak of the COVID-19 pandemic, anxiety and depression prevalence has increased by 25% globally.

The risk of changes in the mental state of the population came mainly from external risk factors, including prolonged lockdowns, social isolation, inadequate or misinterpreted information, loss of income, and acute relationship issues with the rising death toll.

Speaking in psychological terms, the pandemic disturbed our core beliefs.

We were in a time of massive upheaval. There were so many things out of control, such as

- How long will the pandemic last?

- How other people behaved

- What was going to happen in our next communities?

The more unknown the circumstances became, the more I felt anxious, drained, and overwhelmed.

The overwhelming number of ambulance services we heard throughout the day, especially during the night, got us into a spiral of negativity.

But as it got a new routine, in that moment, I decided to focus on the concrete things.

Letting go of our need for certainty and control is a challenge worth embracing. If you feel yourself starting to spin out into negativity or panic, grounding yourself in the present moment can stop the negative spiral.

We 'humans' are social animals. We are hardwired for connection. Isolation and loneliness can exacerbate anxiety and depression and even impact our physical health tremendously.

That's why it is important to stay connected as best as we can and reach out for support when we need it.

- It is important to take breaks from stressful thoughts – to simply enjoy each other's company

- To laugh

- To share stories

We need to focus on the other good things going on in our lives.Social distancing taught me some valid lessons.

- Emotions are contagious. So be wise about whom you turn to for support

- Most of us need reassurance, advice, a pep talk, or a sympathetic ear during difficult times. But we must be careful about who we choose as a sounding board. Avoid people who tend to be very negative or reinforce and ramp up your fears

- Taking care of the body and spirit

- Eating healthily, getting plenty of sleep, and meditating became some of my core habits during the pandemic

- Being kind to yourself

- Make a routine that is as best as you can

- Taking time out for activities you enjoy. Reading a book, watching a comedy, playing a fun board game with family, trying a new recipe, craft, or a piece of art

It doesn't matter what you do as long as it takes you out of worries.

Treat Yourself Well:

Take up a relaxation practice. When stressors throw your nervous system out of balance, relaxation techniques such as deep breathing, meditation, and yoga can bring you back into a state of balance. Regular practice delivers the greatest benefits, so make sure you set aside even a little of your time every day.

The 6 best doctors are sunlight, rest, water, air, food, and exercise. Steve Jobs, in his final speech, said:

You can employ someone to drive the car for you and make money for you, but you cannot bear your sickness for yourself. Material things replaced can be lost or found. But there is one thing that can never be found when it's lost - 'life'.

Chapter 5

SPAM (Surya Namaskar, Pranayama, Affirmations And Meditation) - The Ultimate Health Module

In the era of digitalisation, the internet has made all fitness programmes easily accessible to you from the comfort of your home.

Whether you're thinking about Pilates, yoga, Zumba, or strength training, you will find something online that is new and exciting.

Think of your health as a long road trip. If you miss an exit, would you keep going in the wrong direction? Obviously not. You'd turn around as quickly as possible and get yourself on the right track. Everyone experiences a lack of motivation at some point in their lives. If we are seeking comfort (pleasure) and avoid discomfort (pain), we're going to choose our warm beds. Good health is the most important foundation for any individual to progress.

So make the choice to wake up every single day and give your body the first few hours of the best health.

My SPAM is a complete goodness package. There's only one body, and we need to take care of it. We often neglect our health like SPAM mail. We dump our bodies with junk food and feed our minds with a lot of negative emotions. Before spam can trigger all sorts of negative responses in a critical digital media world, I would like to explain that this abbreviation SPAM will ward off all the procrastination and laziness from you. As we ignore spam in our inbox, let us not ignore our body and mind. The 20-minute module specially created for you can be life-changing in terms of your health and mind. Most of us treat our bodies like trash, leaving them uncared for. So let this word now remind you of the goodness. Let's pledge not to spam our bodies or minds. When you have a high level of well-being, you will also tend to have a confident and go-getting attitude, which will enable you to succeed in all your aspirations. Health insurance is already an astronomically high expense. Constantly being seen by a medical professional will only skyrocket those costs and take money away from achieving your financial goals. Making money takes energy, so healthy energy levels are often necessary. You may also spend a lot of money on sneakers, smoothies, supplements and so on. But having a healthy routine sets apart everything else.

Listen to the rhythm of your body. Start prioritising your needs and keep life very simple.

Stress can build up and grow if not tackled and can often result in us feeling overwhelmed.

Taking time out for yourself is one of the important things you should do in life, yet many of us are trying to juggle everything else.

Allowing yourself to relax and unwind is vital to keep yourself and your mental state intact.

In today's digital age, it's easy to feel overwhelmed by constant notifications and social media updates.

Try setting aside an hour or 2 each day. Use the time to read a book, meditate, take a walk, do some stretches, or simply relax and do nothing.

Taking some time away can help you disconnect from the digital world and reconnect with yourself.

We only tend to worry about ourselves and be anxious when we fall sick.

What if we got into a conscious living? We must value our body and treat it like a temple. As the popular quote doing the rounds on the internet goes, **"You are the books you read, the movies you watch, the people you spend time with, the conversations you engage in."** Choose wisely what you feed into your mind. Very few of us prioritise our wellness and happiness.

Life is busy and crazy, right? Yes, it is. But if we don't take care of our health and wellness, the other aspects will begin to fall apart.

Our mind, body, and soul are all interconnected. Before you can help others, you have to take care of yourself.

Making time for yourself will pave the way for long-term health and vitality. So, put yourself above everyone else. Surround yourself with positivity and wellness.

It's like when you were young, your parents always told you, "Growing up, surround yourself with good people." The same goes for your adult life, health, and wellness.

If you surround yourself with people who will have a positive influence on your well-being, you are going to be better off.

So, spend time with people and environments that constantly promote health and wellness.

Negative people's pessimistic outlook can drag your mood, making you feel sullen and cynical.

Some people are negative simply because they know it can rile you. Learn to counterattack such people with your positivity.

For instance, if your neighbour constantly complains about life, you teach them to count their blessings instead and have an optimistic outlook. When people realise their negativity falls on deaf ears, they may give up on their incessant nagging or complaining habits.

Spam is a good way to reconnect with your body.

These Practices are interlinked with strengths that help you in building a good life. Surya Namskar gives me strength (Strength to endure challenging situations),Pranayama brought in a lot of positivity into my life (as it is proven that breathing improves our mood and is imperial to our mental health) The practice of Affirmation has helped me shape my attitude. Meditation has helped me develop a stronger mindset.

- Surya Namaskar Stands for strength

- Pranayama- Positivity

- Affirmations-Attitude

- Meditation- Mind

So, SPAM it is! It takes 20 minutes (5 minutes of Surya Namaskar, 5 minutes of pranayama, 5 minutes of affirmations and meditations). Starting with this short journey can be a whole lot transformative in terms of building good health and immunity.

So, how are these attributes linked to each practice?

Exercise improves the quality of life. Each one can have their own method of working out. For some, it's the gym, and for some, it's from the comfort of doing things at home.

It's human nature to set and chase goals. However, sometimes goals can also feel daunting, overwhelming, and downright stressful.

Setting Micro-Goals:
I am a big believer in dreaming big. So, when it comes to turning my dreams into reality, I use a self-improvement strategy called micro goal setting that applies to pretty much every aspect of life.

Micro-goals can apply to so many aspects of life, especially in the health and wellness realm.

You can set micro-goals to get

- Stronger

- Get better sleep

- Become more flexible

- Be more positive

Get into conscious living by implementing simple daily practices

What I love about micro-goals is that they are tangible, specific, and task-oriented.

You can think of micro goal setting like running a marathon. To run a marathon, you should set smaller goals, such as jogging one mile or 2 and then perhaps signing up for a 5k race. You certainly don't have to be a runner to put this strategy to work.

No goal is too great when you realise the power of chipping away at it every day, much like the saying progress over perfection.

- Ultimate Goal vs Small Goal

- The ultimate goal - losing 20-30 pounds

- Micro-goals – attending a fitness class and refuelling the body with healthy snacks

- The ultimate goal - finding a job you love

- Micro-goals - To focus on enhancing your best skills

- The ultimate goal - travel around the world

- Micro goal: making a list of must-visit destinations and estimating the money required to visit them

As part of my micro goal setting, I implemented SPAM as part of my daily routines. Sticking to a morning routine is important to me. The morning hours are your magical hours when put to best use. Having a structured yet relaxed morning, especially during weekdays, is something I have always prioritised.

I like the calmness of the mornings, and cultivating a morning routine is the first step to wellness. In Ayurveda, this is called dinacharya.

I indulge in a morning ritual that includes Surya Namaskar, Pranayama, Affirmations, and meditation. Based on the drastic positive changes I've witnessed, if you put these methods into practice, the return on your investment will be there for you to draw on for years to come. If your day allows at least an hour for your morning routine, just commit to it and make it your top priority.

On the days I resist self-care in the mornings (it happens on most days when we lack consistency), I never feel as centred, empowered, and clear as on the days when I start off by honouring the Sacred power within myself through these techniques.

Arising before 6 am helps me feel light and clear. Modern science agrees that syncing our circadian rhythms with nature has many health benefits, including increased immunity and decreased inflammation.

The 4 techniques that I am highlighting may be known to all and are common. 'SPAM', when done together, can have tremendous good results for the body and mind.

Start your journey and explore the goodness!

Surya Namaskar or Sun Salutations:

Surya Namaskar, or sun salutations, are a sequence of 12 powerful yoga poses. Besides being a great cardiovascular workout, Surya Namaskar is known to have an immensely positive impact on the mind and body.

1 set of Surya Namaskar burns 14 calories. 10-15 rounds burn around 150-200 calories. It's one of the most powerful yoga sequences. Practising Surya Namaskar steps is best done early morning on an empty stomach. Each round of sun salutation consists of 2 sets, each set is composed of 12 yoga poses. Besides good health, Surya Namaskar also provides an opportunity to express gratitude to the sun for sustaining life on this planet.

Plenty of Online tutorials are available for doing surya namaskar. you can pick any and practice in perfecting the 12 asanas.

Benefits of Surya Namaskar

1. Helps maintain cardiovascular health.

2. An excellent exercise for weight loss.

3.   Strengthens the immune system

4.   Helps in stretching, flexing, and toning the muscles.

Practising sun salutations every day can give you a range of benefits like a stronger spine, better digestion, and glowing skin.

The key to performing a good sun salutation is giving your 100% in every posture.

For a deeper experience, close your eyes and practice at a slow, rhythmic speed. If you only have 10-15 minutes to spare for your practice, flow through this ancient sequence of yoga postures.

Surya Namaskar is nothing but a breathing meditation.

Through the breathing sequence of inhaling and exhaling, Surya Namaskar oxygenates the blood and helps the circulatory system run properly. This exercise purifies the blood.

Regular practice of Surya Namaskar allows you to feel relaxed and free of anxiety and worry.

In addition, it helps women with regular menstrual cycles. Surya Namaskar can also aid in natural childbirth.

The practice of Surya Namaskar lowers cholesterol levels in the body and increases blood circulation.

When practised at a faster pace, it is a great cardio exercise and a good workout for thighs, abs, and buttocks.

Surya Namaskar in conjunction with a balanced diet and rest will give you a healthy gut and a good immune system.

It helps with problems associated with the lower body, like joint pains and nerve problems.

The forward fold pose in Surya Namaskar helps the digestive system to function efficiently.

Surya Namaskar aims to open our nerve centres or chakras, which are places in our body associated with the different divine or higher energies.

This practice is more relevant for today's world irrespective of gender, geography, religion, or socioeconomic background.

This civilisation of holistic wellness should be passed on to future generations.

In reality, Surya Namaskar is my daily healing balm. It's the most sacred, revered practice of my routine.

I move slowly and deliberately, keeping track of my breath; I watch my inhalation and exhalation.

I also move with vigour at times to awaken my entire system. When soulfully done, it will transcend you beyond time and space. No matter how low you feel in the moment, you will end up recharging yourself with just a few sets and daily rounds.

The first few attempts can feel overwhelming; you may find your body rigid, and you may feel tired after doing 2 rounds. However, by consistently practising for

21 days and getting familiar with the poses, you will start to enjoy it. The Surya Namaskar sequence teaches you so much, not just about yoga poses but yoga as a whole. The more you practice, the more mindful and meditative you become. Even though I regularly walk, Surya Namaskar pulls me out of my sedentary lifestyle. I have never felt guilty about not hitting the gym. Regardless of where you are in your fitness journey, exercising will benefit your daily routine.

Sun salutation is considered the wholesome yoga workout for 'busy bees'.

288 yoga poses in 12 minutes.

One round of sun salutation consists of 12 yoga poses. One set consists of 2 rounds of sun salutation: first stretching the right side of the body and then the left side. So, when you do 12 sets, you are completing 12 x 2 rounds in each set x 12 yoga poses each = 288 yoga poses in 12 to 15 minutes.

There is no other workout as beneficial as Surya Namaskar. Even if you skip the gym or any other form of your regular workout, this can compensate for all that.

It's most effective for weight loss as it involves the whole body.

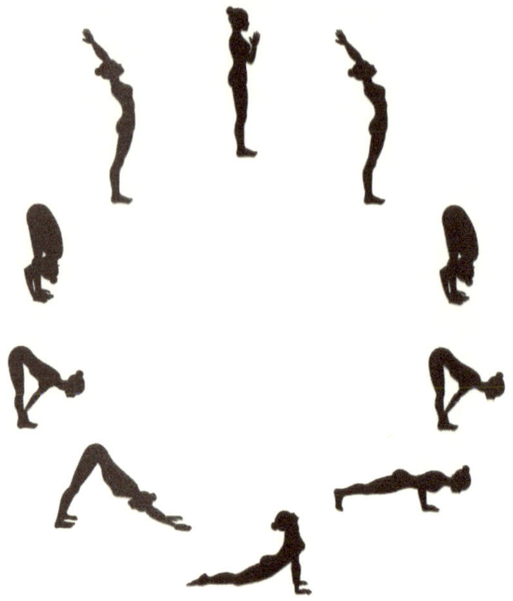

Every discipline cultivates a positive aspect.

Strength:

Building inner strength has been a personal journey for me, shaped by various experiences and deliberate practices over the years. Here are a few key aspects of my journey:

Self-reflection And Awareness:

I started becoming more aware of my thoughts, emotions, and reactions in different situations. This self-reflection helped me understand my strengths, weaknesses, and areas where I needed to improve.

Mindfulness Practice:

I integrated mindfulness into my daily routine, practising meditation and staying present in the moment. Mindfulness has been crucial in managing stress and enhancing my ability to stay calm and focused during challenges and setbacks.

Facing Challenges Head-on:

Instead of avoiding difficulties, I learnt to face them courageously. Each challenge became an opportunity to learn and grow, whether it was navigating personal setbacks or professional obstacles.

Building Resilience Through Adversity:

Adversities have taught me resilience. By reframing setbacks as opportunities for growth and learning, I have been able to bounce back stronger and more determined.

Setting Boundaries And Prioritising Self-care:

Learning to say No when necessary and prioritising my well-being has been essential. Setting boundaries has helped me preserve my energy and maintain a healthy balance in my life.

Seeking Support And Building Relationships:

I've surrounded myself with supportive friends and family who provide encouragement and guidance that I absolutely need at times. Strong relationships have been a source of emotional strength and resilience.

Continuous Learning And Growth:

I embrace a growth mindset, viewing every experience as a chance to learn and improve. Setting goals, both personal and professional, keeps me motivated and focused on continuous self-improvement.

Overall, building inner strength has been a gradual process of self-discovery, resilience building, and personal development. It's about cultivating a strong sense of self, fostering positive habits, and navigating life's challenges with courage and grace.

Pranayama:

Pranayama is the practice of breath regulation. It is a main component of yoga, an exercise for physical and mental well-being.

What exactly is pranayama?

You control the timing, duration, and frequency of every breath. The goal of pranayama is to connect your body and mind. It supplies rich oxygen to your body while removing toxins. One who practices pranayama regularly is able to develop a lustrous face, clarity of voice, brightness of eyes, freedom from diseases like asthma, sinusitis, hypertension, indigestion, and many more.

Pranayama involves different breathing techniques:

- Alternate breathing (Nadishodhana) - alternate nostril breathing, which balances the left and right sides of the brain

- Victorious breathing (Ujayi) - A slow, deep breath with a slight constriction of the throat, creating a soft sound

- Honeybee humming breathing (Brahmari) - it involves producing a humming sound while exhaling

- Bellows breath (Bhastrika) - it is a dynamic pranayama technique characterised by rapid and forceful breathing

- Kapalbhati - A rapid, forceful exhalation followed by passive inhalation to invigorate and cleanse the respiratory system

Pranayama benefits:

- Acts as a stress reliever
- Boosts the immune system
- Treats sleep disorders
- Helps and aids in weight loss
- Improves concentration and focus
- Improves the cardiovascular system
- Reduces the risk of hypertension
- Makes you more aware

Pranayama brings more clarity to the mind and good health to the body. The physical and mental health are intertwined and they are not separate from each other. The greatest indicator of life expectancy is not genetics, diet, or exercise, but lung capacity. With greater lung capacity comes greater longevity and better health.

Pausing to take deep, calm breaths can have an immediate calming effect on the mind and body.

Brahmari Pranayama - BEE Breathing:

Soothe your nervous system, calm restless thoughts and create more focus with this yogic breathing technique.

Method:

- Find a comfortable position
- Gently close off your ears with your fingers
- Inhale deeply through your nose, sensing your abdomen softly rising
- Exhale while making an extended humming sound like HUMMMMMMMM
- Continue the humming sound until you need to take another inhalation. Repeat 3-5 rounds

Sitali Pranayama:

Also known as the cooling breath, sitali is ideal for relaxing the body after an intense day. Regular practice cleanses the body, eliminating toxins, stress, and excess heat from the body.

Step-by-step:

- Sit on your yoga mat with your legs crossed or in the lotus position

- Keep your spine straight. Keep your hands in Gyan Mudra

- Breathe deeply 3 times with an open mouth and exhale through your nose to prepare yourself

- Stick out the tongue and roll it up in the shape of a U

- Inhale through your rolled-up tongue, and towards the end of inhalation, lower your chin to your chest as far as you can. This blocking of the throat is called jalandhara bandha

- In this position, hold your breath for 6 to 8 seconds

Before you exhale, lift your chin up, draw your tongue back, and close your mouth. Now, exhale completely through your nostrils. This completes one round of sitali pranayama.

Nadi Shodhan:

Nadi = subtle energy channel; Shodhan = cleaning, purification; Pranayama = Breathing technique.

Nadis are subtle energy channels in the human body that can be blocked due to various reasons. The Nadi Shodhan Pranayama is a breathing technique that helps clear these blocked energy channels, thus calming the mind. This technique is also called Anulom Vilom Pranayama.

What blocks the nadis?

- Nadis can get blocked due to stress

- Toxicity in the physical body also leads to blockage of nadis

- Unhealthy lifestyle

Method:

- Sit comfortably with your spine erect and shoulders relaxed. Keep a gentle smile on your face

- Place your left hand on the left knee with palms open to the sky or in Chin Mudra

- Place the tip of the index finger and middle finger of the right hand between the eyebrows, the ring finger and little finger on the left nostril, and the thumb on the right nostril. We will use the ring finger and the little finger to open or close the left nostril and the thumb for the right nostril

- Press your thumb on the right nostril and breathe out gently through the left nostril

- Now breathe in from the left nostril and then press the left nostril gently with the ring finger and the little finger. Remove the right thumb from the left nostril, and breathe out from the right

- Breathe in from the right nostril and exhale from the left. You have now completed one round of Nadi Shodhan Pranayama. Continue inhaling and exhaling from alternate nostrils

- Complete 9 such rounds by alternately breathing from both nostrils. After every relaxation, remember to breathe in from the same nostril from which you exhaled. Keep your eyes closed and continue taking such long, deep, and smooth breaths

Bhastrika:

Bhastrika pranayama is the process of rapid inhalation and exhalation, which gives a boost to the body, and hence it is aptly called the yogic breath of fire. So whenever you feel the body needs energy, try Bhastrika Pranayama.

Steps to follow:

- Sit in Vajrasana or Sukhasana

- (Pranayama can be more effective in Vajrasana as your spine is erect and the diaphragmatic movement is better)

- Make a fist and fold your arms, placing them near your shoulders

- Inhale deeply, raise your hands straight up and open your fists

- Exhale slightly forcefully, bring your arms down next to your shoulders and close your fists

- Continue for 20 breaths

- Relax with your palms on your thighs

- Take a few normal breaths

- Continue for 2 more rounds

It's great for energising the body and mind. It helps with sinus, bronchitis, and other respiratory issues.

Ujjayi pranayama: (Victorious breath, perhaps ocean breath)

In this breathing technique, you constrict the back of the throat to support lengthening each breath cycle. Each inhalation and exhalation is long, full, deep, and controlled. It increases oxygen consumption. It's compared to the sound of the wind through the trees or the waves coming to the shore.

Step-by-step:

- Sit up tall with your shoulders relaxed away from your ears and close your eyes

- In ujjayi breathing, both inhalation and exhalation are done through the nose

- As you inhale and exhale, keep your mouth closed

- Constrict your throat to the point that your breathing makes a rushing noise, almost like snoring

- Control your breath with your diaphragm

- Keep your inhalations and exhalations equal in duration

- At first, it may feel like you are not getting sufficient air, but the technique gets easier with practice

Benefits: decreased anxiety, improved concentration, help in managing hypothyroidism.

Kaphalbhati:

Kapalbhati is a powerful breathing exercise in yoga, offering numerous physical and mental benefits. Our breath has amazing recuperative powers.

Steps:

- Sit comfortably with your spine erect. Place your hands on the knees with the palms open to the sky

- Take a deep breath in

- As you exhale, pull your navel back towards the spine. Do as much as you can comfortably. Keep the right hand to feel the abdominal muscles contract

- As you relax the navel and abdomen, the breath flows into your lungs automatically

- Take 25 such breaths to complete one round of Kapal Bhati

- Do a few more rounds

- The exhalation in Kapal Bhati is active and forceful. So just throw out your breath

- Keep your awareness on breathing out. The inhalation will automatically happen naturally when you relax your abdominal muscles

- Practice this technique at home on an empty stomach

It comes with enormous health benefits such as enhancing the capacity of the lungs and making them stronger, energising the nervous system and rejuvenating the brain cells, improving blood circulation and adding radiance to the face, and calming and uplifting the mind.

Chapter 6

Breathing Framework

The way we breathe has changed over time. Babies are expert breathers; no one had to teach them to breathe. If you look closer, they breathe into their little bellies. But over time, this changes; kids stop breathing into the belly and start to be chest breathers, and that's what most adults do. Our breathing pace, intensity, and duration impact us on a physiological, mental, emotional, and spiritual level.

Two functions in the human body are contrast and involuntary.

1. The beating of the heart and

2. Breathing

By becoming conscious of our breathing and infusing our normal breath with our own light of consciousness, we can evolve multi-dimensionally.

Facts pertaining to breath:

*   Shortness of breath results in a short lifespan; unconscious breathing is typically at a high rate and results in a shorter lifespan

- That's why smaller creatures such as cats, dogs, and squirrels breathe more rapidly and have shorter lifespans

- Dogs breathe aggressively; on the other hand, elephants, tortoises, and larger mammals breathe much slower and live longer

Breathwork or mindfulness:

- Practising any form of breathwork is deeply integrative, connecting, and a restorative experience

- Every time you do deep breathwork, you might feel a deeper connection with yourself

- Peace is radiating through your mind and body

- A sense of oneness

- You will experience gentleness, tension release, and other calming sensations

- Breathwork is done in many different ways. Some form of breathing is practised widely everywhere

- In schools, yoga studios, therapy, sports, holistic healing, nursing, meditation, and trauma healing. In breathing, picking up the cues is important. Listen to your body's cues and if a certain style is not right for you. If a particular technique feels uncomfortable, then close out that practice and adopt a new one that feels easier and more convenient

As you get the hang of each technique, you can keep adding other elements and combinations that will contribute to your practice.

- How many breaths have you taken this minute?

- What is the intention of your practice today?

- How are you feeling mentally, emotionally, and physically?

Using Breath To Develop Consciousness:
- The first step in learning to breathe is to consciously develop an intimate awareness of our own breathing

- The first step in practice is to count each inhalation and exhalation

- Sit in a comfortable posture

- Count each time you inhale and exhale

- Observe your breathing pattern intently

- Count each complete breath (inhalation + exhalation) until you reach 20 counts, and then reverse the counting from 20 to 0

There are numerous breathing techniques. I would like to highlight a few practices that i personally follow as part of my daily rituals.

1. Diaphragmatic breathing

2. Box breathing (4:4:4)

3. Straw breath

4. Candle breath

When I have trouble sleeping, I count my own breath and try to relax.

You are constantly breathing, so you can choose to focus on it at any given time, any place.

Conscious breathing can be done:

- While commuting to work
- At work, before meeting your deadlines
- While watching television
- When you have absolutely nothing else to do
- The rhythm and the rate of our breathing also vary with our emotional patterns
- Happy and overwhelmed
- Angry, anxious, stressed, or startled
- Sleeping (relaxed state)
- Physical exertion or when experiencing any pain

For the most part, we don't notice the regular ebb or flow of breathing. We often fail to notice the powerful, portable, and transformative process of mindfulness and breathing.

Having an awareness of breathing can shift from the monkey mind of thinking to a calm place of rhythm and flow.

Coming out of stress, filled with an overthinking brain and giving you a few moments to slow down and calm, is good medicine for the body and soul.

When you watch your breath, you are more aware of your present.

- Our world pulsates with patterns and rhythms
- Eyelids flutter
- Hearts beat
- Lungs breathe
- Movement, rhythm, and patterns sustain the life of energy. So, conscious breathing stimulates the force of life energy
- Through constant practice of breathing, fuel your mind and body

Practice:

Take a deep breath and expand your belly. PAUSE (hold your breath for a few seconds). Exhale slowly to the count of 5.

Congratulations, you have just calmed your nervous system.

For centuries, yogis have used breath control/ pranayama to promote concentration and improve vitality. Buddha advocated breath meditation as a

- **Breath**
- **Inhale**
- **Hold**
- **Exhale (Repeat)**

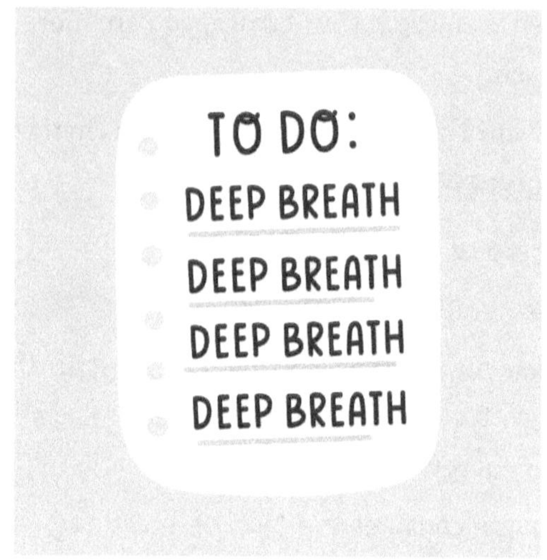

Diaphragmatic Breathing:

When you breathe normally, you don't use your lungs to their full capacity. The diaphragm is a large muscle that sits below the lungs and helps the lungs expand and contract.

Normal breathing is relatively shallow. Diaphragmatic breathing is a deep breathing exercise that fully engages the diaphragm and increases the efficiency of the lungs.

Follow the instructions below:

- Lie down on a flat surface with a pillow under your head, or sit in a comfortable position

- Place one hand on the middle of the upper chest

- Place the other hand on the stomach

- Inhale slowly, breathe in through the nose, drawing the breath down to the stomach

- The stomach should push upward against the hand while the chest remains still

- To exhale, tighten the abdominal muscles and let the stomach fall downward while exhaling through the pursed lips. Again, the chest should remain still

This breathing exercise can be practised for 5-10 minutes around 2-3 times each day to ensure you are engaged in conscious breathing throughout the day.

Once you become comfortable with diaphragmatic breathing, you can do this practice anywhere, even while seated or standing.

While practising diaphragmatic breathing, it is important to keep the head, neck, and shoulders relaxed.

Benefits:
- Improves the lung functioning capacity

- Improves cognitive functioning

- Lowers blood pressure

- Reduces stress and anxiety

- Improved chronic breathing conditions

Breathing Facts:

An average adult inhales and exhales about 11,000 litres of air per day while resting.

Every emotion is connected to our breath. If you can change the breath, change the rhythm, you can change the emotion.

The vagus nerve is the longest nerve in your body. It connects your brain to many important organs throughout the body, including the gut, heart, and lungs.

The Vagus nerve helps to relax and destress.

How to Activate:
- **Deep, slow breathing**
- **Meditation**
- **Exercise**

A few minutes of breathing, can energise the body and mind.

Strengthen the Lungs:

With diaphragmatic breathing, you are allowing more air into your lungs, and your body immediately switches to a relaxed state.

- Observe your breath and note if it's deep or shallow
- Chest breathing is shallow, which signals stress to the brain

- Abdominal breathing boosts respiration, supplies a rich amount of oxygen, and signals that all is well

- The Nobel Prize winner and American pharmacologist Louis Ignarro has said that

- Nasal breathing releases nitric oxide. What does nitric oxide do?

- It directly interacts with viruses to kill them

- Bhramari increases nitric oxide 15 times more in the nasal passages

Box Breathing Technique:

Box breathing technique, also referred to as square breathing, is a deep restorative technique. Box breathing is a simple but powerful relaxation technique.

It is very easy and quick to learn. Anyone can practise this technique, and it is extremely helpful in stressful situations. It is the best practice for recentering oneself.

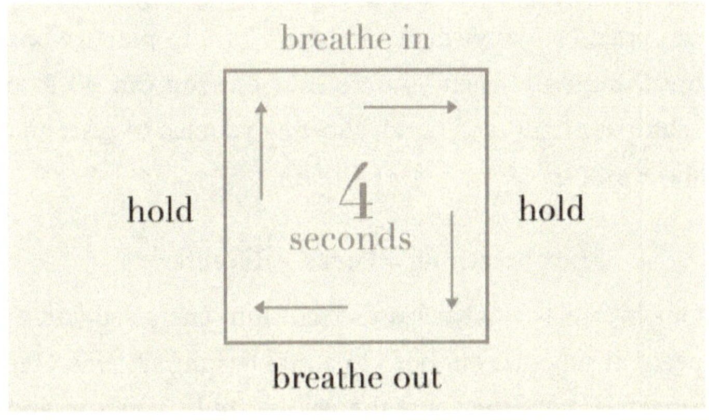

FOUR STEPS TO MASTER BOX BREATHING:

- Step 1: Breathe in, counting to 4 (1, 2, 3, 4) steadily and slowly. Feel the air enter your lungs

- Step 2: Hold your breath for 4 seconds. Avoid inhaling or exhaling for 4 seconds

- Step 3: breathe out for 4 seconds. Exhale

Repeat this exercise as many times as you can. This exercise can help you cope with panic attacks and stress when feeling overwhelmed.

Benefits:

- Helps you to refocus when you are having a busy or stressful day. Eases panic, worry, and anxiety

- Keeps you calm while preparing for your day

- Lowers cortisol, a stress hormone that can improve your mood

One of the biggest advantages of box breathing is that you can practice it anywhere. You don't have to practice box breathing only when you are stressed. You can do it to calm your body and mind, allowing yourself to reset and stay fresh.

Box breathing = Focus + Recentering

Our breath is what helps us feel calm, energised and at peace. It supports our body's natural healing systems. Our breath is more than just the air we are bringing in and out of our body. Celebrate the joy of breathing for every moment you live.

The Straw Breath:

The straw breath is a perfect way to neutralise any stagnant energies. Straw breath is one of the best ways to equalise oxygen coming in and the rate of carbon dioxide going out.

The keys to this breath are to keep your inhalations and exhalations at the same pace, duration, and intensity.

Note: If you have any history of fainting, panic attacks, or vertigo from taking quick breaths, then this won't be right for you.

Activity:

- Sit or stand comfortably upright
- Take 3 medium sips of air through your mouth as if you were sipping water through a straw
- Blow out at the same pace 3 times from your mouth as if you were blowing out of a straw
- Repeat for a few rounds all the way up to 7 minutes
- Tip: It's fun to use an actual straw for this technique. Reusable straws are perfect for this practice
- Benefits: increased energy levels, increased feel-good hormones; improved digestion, improved respiration, releases stagnant energy from the body, a great stress reliever

Candle Breath for Energy:

This technique is very similar to blowing out candles on the cake. This technique is a good one if you are someone who keeps sitting all day at work.

The movements of this breathing technique will activate your chest and belly.

Method:

- You can practise this technique in any position
- Breathe in through your mouth
- Blow out air from your mouth as if you are blowing out a candle
- On those inhales, breathe into the belly and chest at the same time, filling up most of your body with air at once
- On those exhales, squeeze your belly so that you are releasing all the air from your body at once
- Repeat at least 5 times

Benefits:

- Increased energy
- Relieves stress
- Improves focus and concentration

The humming breath:

- The humming breath or brahmari is an absolute way to bring peace and calm to yourself. This breathwork has an exceptional element to it: its vibrational healing

Benefits:

- Relieves stress

- Relaxes your body

- Relieve your nervousness

- Improves the quality of your sleep

- Improves concentration and focus

The practice:

- Sit or stand with a comfortably straight spine

- Closed eyes are recommended for this practice

- Breathe in through your nose into your full body for at least 5 seconds

- With your mouth closed, hum as if you are saying "HMMM" until you are out of breath

- Repeat as many times as you like

- Try this practice in a group. The collective humming sound will have a superb healing effect on your nervous system

Breathwork: I am love & light:

I AM LOVE AND LIGHT

As you inhale, visualise clean healing energy entering your body and filling you with vitality and strength.

As you exhale, visualise any tension or negative energy leaving your body, allowing yourself to feel more relaxed and at peace.

Repeat the mantra: I am love and light.

Reflecting on my personal experience with pranayama, I have noticed several shifts in my perspective and well-being.

Initially, I found it challenging to focus on my breath and struggled with different techniques. I gradually evolved over time and observed good progress in my ability to control my breath, which in turn improved my overall well-being. Pranayama helped me cultivate a deeper sense of tranquillity. I was more present in my daily activities and able to concentrate better. I also experienced increased energy levels and vitality.

A greater sense of inner peace, improved self-awareness, and a more positive outlook became a part of my life all too naturally.

Positivity and Perspective Are Key to Leading a Good, Healthy Life:

Being authentic these days is kind of hard to achieve. We are constantly bombarded with what we should be doing with our lives. It is rightly said that a healthy mind leads to a healthy life.

When you focus on positive thoughts, your brain releases neurotransmitters that promote feelings of happiness, contentment, and well-being.

Positive thinking can be very challenging to put into practice.

Creator Charisse Glenn's work is based on a fourfold philosophy:

- **The happier we are, the kinder we become**
- **One power lies in how we react to things that are out of control**
- **We can change ourselves at any given point in life**
- **Life starts with the first step**

"Pleasure, comfort, gratitude, hope, and inspiration are catalysts that increase our happiness and help us lead a joyous and fulfilling life."

In today's fast-paced world, it is very common to feel stressed or worried. From children to adults, everyone is bearing some challenges.

Children dread examinations.

Adults face so many pressures, including working, running the family, paying bills, etc.

Nobody can remain optimistic 365 days a year. The minute you are faced with a challenge, you tend to get caught in the spiral of negativity.

A good technique to use when you notice yourself getting flustered or weighed down with negativity - PAUSE.

Take a moment to focus your awareness on the present and breathe deeply while paying attention to your 5 senses. This is called the grounding technique.

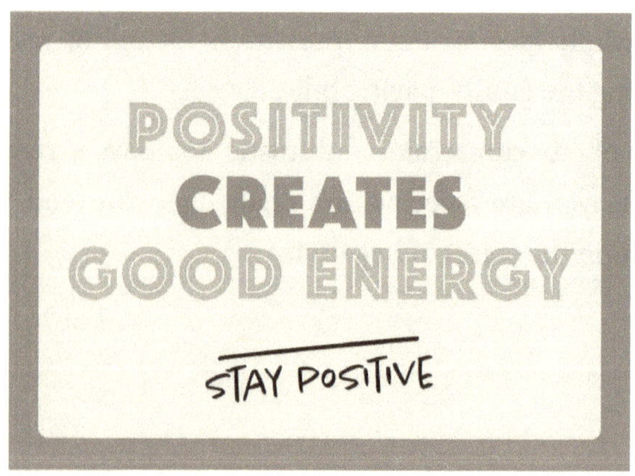

Small yet impactful actions such as:

Practising gratitude

Finding joy in simple pleasures and maintaining a positive mindset contribute to overall well-being. Practice positivity, and everything else will fall into place.

<u>Four ways to bring good into your world:</u>

- Happiness – seek purpose, not possessions
- Compassion – have empathy for others
- Gratitude – Appreciate the little things
- Calm - create your own serenity

Emotions are a natural part of life, and they play an important role in our physical and mental health.

In shaping future generations, it is important for parents and educators to understand how to help children and young people manage their emotions in a healthy way.

By understanding and managing their emotions in a healthy way, children and young people develop into happy and well-adjusted adults.

Positivity does not just happen with reading self-help books, attending discourses, or meditation.

The mind is a very powerful place, and every time a negative thought flashes in your mind, you can snap yourself out of it.

Negative thoughts aren't always a bad thing. Acknowledging that you made a mistake gives you a chance to reflect on it. Positivity neither comes easily nor naturally, you require a lot of persistence and hard work.

Negativity is laziness. It takes a lot of work to remain positive, but positivity always pays off.

It is easy to end up in a bad mood when we face adversity. It is hard to stay positive when faced with our own problems. It can get even harder when we are living through everyday frustrations.

Common scenarios that bog our energy down include arguments at the workplace, rough situations within the family, and gloomy days with friends. These are some of the encounters that can adversely impact our minds often and reflect on our mood. Because we tend to care for the people around us, we become susceptible to negativity. It is important to keep our sanity intact.

Exercise:
- Close your eyes for a few minutes. Inhale and exhale deeply
- Inhale positivity, Exhale negativity
- Inhale calmness, Exhale tensions
- Inhale joy, Exhale anger
- Inhale acceptance, Exhale worries
- Inhale peace, Exhale anxiety
- Inhale silence, Exhale Inner noise

- Inhale Gratitude, Exhale ungratefulness
- This is a sure way to invite positive feelings into your thoughts

If you hear someone constantly complaining, allow them to vent for a few minutes. But if you find someone complaining all the time, and if you find yourself agreeing with them, then you are holding yourself responsible for reinforcing that behaviour in them. Instead, be wise enough to offer an alternate solution. Sometimes, problems can be overwhelming, which makes it tempting to crawl under the sheet and cover yourself away from the world.

Imagine losing your loved one or job or having a serious illness striking you. These can be some of the life-altering situations. Instead of trying to suppress or ignore negative emotions, we should acknowledge and validate them, allowing ourselves to fully experience them.

When someone comes to us with problems or is going through a tough time, we should practise empathy and active listening. We should focus on realistic positivity, which means acknowledging both the good and the bad in a situation.

In the era of digitalisation, positivity can seem daunting. It's hard sometimes to resist the urge to go down the rabbit hole of negativity.

I follow people who uplift my spirits.

I follow pages and content that align with my values and morality. This is one of the best ways I avoid any form of negativity.

Affirmations:

- By using the power of positive affirmations, we can rewire our thinking, foster a positive outlook and align our actions with our dreams

- Hardships, heartbreak, and setbacks are all part of life. From facing difficult relationships, unfulfilling jobs to financial challenges, it's quite easy to feel disheartened

- But that isn't true. Amidst all such challenges, there is a powerful tool that can help change our mindset and manifest a life that we truly desire:

That's called Affirmations.

Whatever we believe becomes true for us. If you face a sudden financial crisis, then on some level, you may believe you are unworthy of being comfortable with money.

If you believe that nothing good ever lasts, maybe you believe that life is out to get you.

If you feel you are unable to attract a relationship, then you may believe nobody loves you enough.

If you have poor health, you may believe illness runs in the family.

Financial disaster———————— I don't attract money.

No friend—————————-I am not loved enough by people.

Problem with work——————— I am not good enough

People pleasing ——————— I always have to do things for others.

Whatever the problem may be, it comes from a thought pattern that later forms into a strong belief system.

Ask yourself, what kind of thoughts do I have to create this? You are never stuck in life. You are only stuck with your thoughts and beliefs. It doesn't matter how long you have had a negative thought pattern, illness, or poor relationship.

We can begin to make a positive shift from today. You are the ultimate power in the world. You get to have whatever you choose to think. Our minds create our future. Whenever we have something that is undesirable, we must use our minds to the best of our ability to change the situation.

We can begin to change it from this very second. I start my day with a daily set of affirmations, setting the highest intention for my health. They work like magic for me. Regardless of how I feel, I quickly decide to take my day in control.

I got into the practice of affirming in the mornings after reading Louise Hay's book You Can Heal Your Life.

In the 1970s, Hay was diagnosed with irreversible cervical cancer, and as a result, she began looking into medical healing alternatives.

Through affirmations and other alternative approaches like positive thinking, she argued we have the power to transform our lives and health.

In later interviews, she lived to the age of 90. She shared how her belief led to the cure of her disease. After reading and researching a lot about affirmations, I decided to make them part of my morning routine.

Before doing affirmations, I would consider going to the doctor even for minor health complaints such as a cold, sore throat, and headaches. But ever since I started putting some positive statements into practice, I have seen a drastic change and results in terms of my health.

My all-time favourite is the one from YouTube by Alena Foxx **for health and immunity**.

- I am grateful for my strong and healthy immune system
- Thank you for my perfect health
- I am healthy and full of energy
- I make healthy choices
- I love to nourish my body by eating healthily

- My immune system is powerful and strong
- Today, I choose to be healthy
- I love myself, and I choose to create a body that heals me
- I choose to remain in a positive state so that my body can heal itself
- Every cell in my body vibrates with optimal health and energy
- I am wrapped in the loving energy of the universe
- I am growing healthier and stronger every single day
- I am healthy and full of energy
- Healing vibrations pulsate through my being, protecting me from all disharmonies
- My body heals quickly and easily
- My body is powerful, and it knows how to heal itself
- I am energetic and grateful for my life
- I now release blockages and lower vibrations from my body and my energetic field
- I have an abundance of health, energy, and vitality
- I am in perfect health
- I enjoy existing in a natural state of well-being
- I am a magnet for uplifting, healthy, and empowering energy
- My body is strong and healthy
- My immune system is strong and healthy

- I trust that I am always protected

- I am a radiant being filled with love and light

- Every single cell of my body is filled with love and light

- Thank you for my perfect health

Affirmations work as a tool for shifting your mindset and achieving your goals, but they are not a magic bullet for instant success or healing.

How do we visualise challenging situations in a positive way?

For example, you might replace a negative or anxious thought like:

"I am so terrible at interviews. I am probably not even as qualified as the other candidate."

Replace the statement with a positive affirmation.

"I have all the necessary skills and experience, and I am the perfect candidate for the job."

Consider that nosy coworker who always asks questions about your personal life. You don't want to say anything to offend, but you also have no intention of answering their questions.

An affirmation like "I can remain calm even when I feel annoyed" might guide you to a habit of deep breathing or grounding exercises when you start to feel agitated.

Affirmations are like planting seeds in the ground.

First, they germinate, then they sprout roots, and then they poke their first little shoots up through the ground. It will take some time to go from a seed to a fully grown plant.

I remember the day I stumbled across a video about affirmations. When I started saying affirmations every single morning, I started sensing some positive shifts taking place in my life.

Slowly but surely, my outlook on life changed for the better. I now have so many wonderful opportunities. If you feel stuck in the same place for too long, perhaps you need to change the way you talk to yourself.

I bet you will have nothing to lose except this old version of yourself that you cling onto because you're comfortable.

It takes a minimum of 21 days to form a brand-new belief or habit.

Remember that you are abundant, powerful, and limitless.

Affirmations can be used for every aspect of life. They can be separated into 5 sections:

- Affirmations for health and wellness

- Success

- Self-love

- Financial abundance and a millionaire mindset

- Morning gratitude

One simple yet profound way to improve mental health is to practice positive affirmations regularly.

Helpful Tips:
- Use the word I am
- Keep it very brief and specific
- Use the present tense
- Include at least one emotion/feeling
- Visualise affirmations
- You can use affirmations to enhance all areas of your life:

Affirmations to Gain Perspective:
- I allow life to unfold
- Clarity will come to me at the right time
- I release all my worries
- I trust that the right answers will come to me at the right time
- I release the need to control outcomes

Affirmations on Self-Confidence:
- I am confident in my abilities
- I am capable of achieving anything I set my mind to
- I am the creator of my own reality
- I am worthy of great success
- I trust that my intuition will lead me to the right path

Affirmations for Body Image:

- I honour my body's need for rest and rejuvenation
- I choose moments that feel good and energising
- I celebrate my body and all it represents
- I am comfortable and confident in my own skin
- I radiate positivity and inspire others
- My body is beautiful, and I carry it with pride
- I trust and listen to my body's wisdom
- I embrace my body with love and self-assurance

Money:

- I am financially abundant
- I am a money magnet
- Money flows freely to me and through me
- I am in harmony with the energy of money
- I am abundant in all areas of my life
- I am connected to the endless abundance of the universe
- I create limitless prosperity by doing what I love
- I am worthy of financial security

Goals:

- I am open to receiving all the blessings of this abundant universe
- I believe in myself and my abilities to achieve goals

- I have a routine that supports my goals

- I stay centred and focused on my goals

- I think clearly and focus on steps for success

- I am consistent, and it shows the desired results

Happiness:

- I choose to be happy at any given moment

- I appreciate all the little things in my life

- I am worthy of feeling happy

- I have everything that I need to be happy

- I am in charge of my own happiness

Love:

- I love myself, and I allow myself to be fully loved

- I am grateful for the love that is around me

- I attract loving relationships into my life

- I am a magnet for healthy and long-lasting friendships

- I am open to giving and receiving love freely and authentically

Peace:

- I am present within myself

- I am grounded, worthy, and whole

- I release what no longer serves me

- I choose peace and serenity

- I inhale peace and exhale worry
- I am at peace with who I am
- I invite peace into every corner of my being
- My heart is a place of tranquillity and harmony
- I breathe in calmness and exhale chaos
- In stillness, I find my strength
- I embrace silence and find serenity within its depths

Self-worth:
- I am proud of myself and my achievements
- I am free of all limiting thoughts and beliefs
- I honour my individual journey, and I am enough just as I am
- I am worthy of kindness, respect, and compassion
- I am a beacon of love and positivity

Wake-up Affirmations
- Today is going to be incredible
- I choose happiness today
- I am grateful for my body
- I am grateful for the new day
- I am the architect of my life
- I attract positive energies into my life
- I am connected to an infinite source
- I create my reality with my thoughts

- I am constantly attracting wealth

- I can conquer anything

- The sunrise fills me with energy

- I have everything I need to make today a great day

- I choose to speak to myself with love and kindness today and always

Bedtime Affirmations:

- I end this day with a positive feeling

- I did the best I could today

- I feel calm and peaceful

- I close my eyes with a grateful heart; tomorrow brings a fresh start

- I am allowing myself to rest peacefully

Affirmations to Feel Good:

- I trust the timing of my life

- I fully trust my intuition

- I feel abundant

- I feel at peace

- I feel happy

- I matter, and my energy is needed in this world

- I love my life

- I am enough just as I am

Affirmations For Clear Skin:

- My skin is always glowing
- My skin Is Perfect
- My skin is naturally radiant
- I attract clear skin effortlessly
- My skin is clear and bright
- My skin is beautiful
- I am grateful for my clear skin
- My skin is like glass
- I attract glowing skin naturally
- My skin is smooth and blemish-free

Weight Loss Affirmations:

- I am patient with my mind and body
- I am well-maintained and fit
- I always care for my body
- I am strong in mind and body
- I love myself and love the shape of my body
- I am leading a healthy lifestyle
- I deserve to be healthy and fit
- I exercise and take good care of my body
- I am so grateful to have a healthy body
- I am completely focused on my health
- I love my energy

- I have vibrant health
- With each passing day, my body is becoming healthier and more energetic

Affirmations for Anxiety:

- I am safe and in control
- I release my worries and embrace calm
- I trust in my ability to handle challenges
- I am worthy of peace and tranquillity
- I choose to focus on the present moment
- I let go of what I cannot control
- I am stronger than my fears
- My mind is clear, and my heart is at peace
- I breathe in peace and exhale tension
- I embrace uncertainty with courage
- I am grounded, centred and calm
- I trust the process of life
- I choose peace over worry
- My body and mind are relaxed and at ease

Pause And Reflect For A Moment Of Gratitude:

- I am grateful for my life
- I am grateful for the love that surrounds me
- I am grateful for being able to learn, grow, and evolve

- I am grateful for every moment that has brought me here

- I am grateful for my ability to choose how I view the world

- I am grateful for the people who love and care for me

- I choose to acknowledge my blessings every day

Affirmations for Manifestations:

- Magic will always surround me

- I can see the future that I want to have and know that it is on its way

- The universe is bringing good things my way, and I am already thankful for them

- I have enough. I do enough. I am enough

- All I need is within me

- I accept myself unconditionally

- I attract massive amounts of happiness

- I have plenty of time and energy to do the things I love to do

- I attract love, success, freedom, and health into my life

- Money is an unlimited resource and is always flowing my way

- I am in the right place at the right time

- Good opportunities will always find me

Every day is a good day. Every day, as soon as you wake up, affirm:

- I welcome love, opportunities, health, happiness, peace, success, inspiration, fulfilment, purpose, gratitude, empowerment, and all that is good for me and my life

As you start to create a new reality for your life based on the words you speak to yourself and the actions you take, watch your life unfold in beautiful ways.

Be compassionate, speak kind words and spread this world with gracious love and much-needed positive energy.

Affirmations have greatly shaped my attitude:

It's been said that attitude is everything. Victor Frankl was a prisoner of war in Germany during World War II at Auschwitz. His mother, father, and brother were all killed in the camp. He had lost everything. He said, "Everything can be taken from man but one thing: the last of human freedoms to choose one's attitude in any given set of circumstances, to choose one's way."

Attitudes are not caused by people or circumstances. We can overcome any situation with a good attitude.

"What is the difference between an obstacle and an opportunity? Our attitude towards it. Every opportunity has a difficulty, and every difficulty has an opportunity." - Sid Low Baxter

I've seen myself go out of the way and do more for people who have a great attitude towards life. People who are humble, joyous, excited, nice, and genuine have more to offer.

I have also seen people who are not so optimistic (selfish, miserable, irritable, sad). They tend to lose out on a lot of experiences because of how they react to situations.

How they become angry too quickly.

How they do not say thank you, sorry, or please

How they take other people for granted.

Within the realm of a great attitude comes gratitude. We should be grateful for everything we have and thank the universe or God for bestowing us with so many blessings.

Benefits of a good or positive attitude:

- Increased productivity

- Better coping skills

- Better resilience

- Enhanced psychological health

Exercise:

- You can examine your attitude with the following questions:

- Do I have beneficial, positive relationships?

- How do I start my day? Do I have a routine that promotes positive energy all day?

- Am I aware of the state of mind and its changes? If I am in a negative state of mind, am I able to change it?

- Is my living space a positive environment? If not, what can I do to make it a positive environment?

- At any given moment, your attitude can be that of a creator or a victim. The first step you need to take to shift from victim mode to creator mode is to take responsibility

Here's the attitude of the creator:

- **I am the creator of my life**

- **I am responsible for myself**

- **I am in charge of my destiny**

Our attitude can be altered through our habits. Today, young people are living through one of the biggest transformations of all time - the rapid digitalisation of society.

We are stuck in a stream of continuous notifications, messages, and a never-ending loop of videos and refreshing newsfeeds, all of which cause constant stress and anxiety.

The digital world can foster a culture of comparison, where we're constantly measuring ourselves against the carefully crafted images of others.

The compounding effects of COVID-19, the climatic crisis, natural disasters, wars, and economic downturns have intensified.

If you truly want to know yourself, turn off your internet, TV, or any other source of entertainment. Go to a quiet place and spend a little time all by yourself. This is where you will end up meeting your real self. This is where you will learn what's truly important to you.

Silence helps bring us back to the place of rest and clarity within, away from the noise of the world.

Keeping a good attitude amidst all the challenges and changes is one of the keys to having a happy and healthy life.

Meditation:

"Meditation provides the nervous system a rest that is 5 times deeper than sleep." - Dr. Mark Hyman

I am an avid meditator. You learn to meditate by meditating. There are no shortcuts to it. The silence and stillness you experience in meditation naturally teach you to go deeper into it.

My first foray into meditation happened when I was in college. I started adopting a daily meditation practice. Now, it has been more than a decade of intense practice.

Meditation, to me, is like breathing. Meditation, like breathing, can be essential for well-being and a natural way to bring calm and clarity into one's life. Meditation Practices can be deeply grounding and integral to maintaining balance.

Anyone who's new to meditation in the beginning can easily tend to feel frustrated or bored.

When starting out, it can be hard to know if you're doing it right.

Practical tips:

- For beginners, a book or a phone app like Headspace or Calm are good options

- Explore different meditation techniques to find the best practice that suits you (mantra meditation, guided, Transcendental, Vipassana, kriya, loving-kindness)

- Some of the differences in meditation techniques can be subtle, yet the difference they make can be significant

Benefits of doing meditation:

- Reduces stress and anxiety

- Regular meditation improves your physical health

- It is beneficial to your body as much as it is beneficial to your mind

- Meditation elevates your mood and emotional state

- It improves your immune system function

- It sharpens focus and improves concentration. (Think of meditation as a gym for your brain)

- Meditation helps you fall into a deep, restorative sleep

Meditation can activate the Vagus nerve, which helps the body shift from a stress response to a relaxation response. The word vagus means wanderer because the vagus nerve literally wanders all over the body, starting from the brain. It is the longest nerve in the body and one of the most important as it sends commands to and takes information from numerous organs, including the heart and gut. The vagus nerve can be thought of as a superhighway that represents the mind-body connection. It also connects the heart, liver, spleen, gall bladder, lungs, neck, ears, and tongue. So, try meditation for a few minutes to stimulate your vagus nerve.

'Meditation is for everyone', whether young or old, try your hand at it. There is no better way to recharge your soul than meditation.

If you can spare a minute per day, start there. Eventually, you may try for 3, 4, and 5 minutes; it's about gradually increasing the time limit. Slowly raise your bars to 10, 20, and 30. Initially, what would have felt too long, with practice, would have passed by in a jiffy. Even half an hour feels less or inadequate for me with practice, like the old adage 'practice makes a man perfect'.

The joy of meditation often comes from the sense of inner peace and clarity.

It provides space to disconnect from the daily stressors and reconnect with oneself. Many find joy in the simplicity of being present and in the gradual unveiling of a deeper sense of calm and contentment. You cannot ignore the power of small steps. While trekking, every step counts, and it pushes you to your final destination.

Once you get the hang of it, meditation will blow your mind.

The average young person approximately checks their Instagram account at least 100 times a day. They remain glued to their mobiles to constantly keep themselves updated on their surroundings. That's how the applications are designed. Our mind seeks entertainment. It craves importance. You wait for stimulation such as a vacation or party or anything that gives you some pleasure.

If you want to ideally break these patterns of momentary pleasure, you must start your journey somewhere someday, and that journey is about seeking yourself.

Exploring meditation is like going beyond your routine.

The mind likes to chatter away. The mind constantly keeps replaying something.

What we said or discussed over dinner last night, stressing over the work deadlines, fretting over an imaginary argument, it is from this superficial level of mind that we spend each day. But under the surface, the mind goes much deeper. While our rush-rush conscious mind sits above the surface, chattering away, our deep mind is always below – seeing, hearing, feeling, taking it all in.

While our conscious mind always wants to be in some other place or time, our deep mind stays present, forever anchored in the here and now.

Conscious mind is always rationalising, judging, fearing, worrying – our deep mind is always cool, calm and collected.

Meditation opens access to everything beneath the surface.

Meditation replaces the scattered, unaware, absent-minded, anxious, depressed, irrational, addicted brain and awakens the person to remain more present, calm, centred, focused, balanced, creative, intuitive, insightful, and highly aware.

Our highest and best self-resides under the surface. People new to meditation often come into the practice with certain assumptions.

They often expect the mind to be completely free of thoughts or the body to automatically enter into a trance-like state.

Well, the reality is these things don't happen overnight; these things do happen more and more as our meditation skills sharpen.

Meditation isn't just about stopping thoughts from entering our mind; it isn't about magically entering a deep, relaxed state; it is more about becoming at ease with our mind and comfortable with our thoughts as they are.

Misconceptions of Meditation:

You can't think or let your mind wander. TRUTH: Thoughts will come. Allow them to. They will quiet down on their own over time.

You have to sit for 20 minutes straight. Truth: Even as little as one minute, when practised regularly, will add up. Begin where you are!

You have to meditate every day. TRUTH: While that's optimal, skipping a day here and there won't hurt. Be gentle with yourself.

Spiritual experiences mean you're progressing. Truth: Meditation is a daily practice, and attaching to special experiences can actually hinder your committed practice.

If you are a mind chatterer the whole time, nothing is happening: TRUTH is even if nothing feels different while you are meditating; your time off the cushion is slowly changing.

Keep showing up!

Exercise:

One Minute Meditation:

- Take a deep breath
- Breathe in through the nose,
- Breathe out through the mouth
- Breathe in, feeling the lungs expanding,
- Breathe out, feeling a sense of letting go

- Breathe in to feel the body getting fuller,

- Breathe out to feel the release of any tension

- Breathe in, feeling alive and awake,

- Breathe out, feeling the muscles relaxing

- Breathe in that sense of fullness,

- Breathe out that unnecessary tension

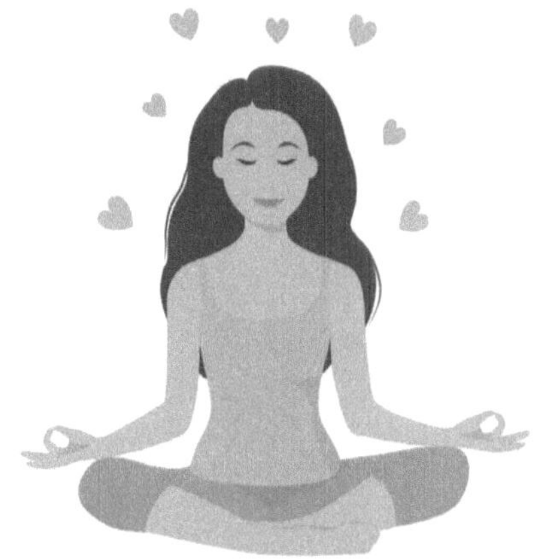

1-minute Meditation:

Close your eyes and bring your awareness to your breath. As thoughts keep arising, imagine them as bubbles. Visualise each one floating away as soon as they appear; be mindful and keep returning to your breath.

Meditation, when combined with nostril breathing (deep inhalations and exhalations) and repeating a mantra, instantly calms the mind.

Mantra Meditation:

Many meditation practitioners believe the vibrations and harmony of chanting certain syllables can enable a deeper meditative state. Repeating a mantra while meditating can also help you find a natural breathing rhythm.

Matching your breath to your mantra can make this process easier and help you feel more relaxed at the same time.

A common and my most favourite mantra is 'OM'. Aum or Om is believed to be the universal sound.

When you chant 'om', both your mind and body are energised, and you tend to feel positive.

Chanting Aum with devotion and a pure heart can lead to a spiritual journey.

Benefits Of Chanting Om:
- Calms the mind
- Reduces stress and anxiety
- Improves focus and attention
- Balances emotions
- Improves sleep quality
- Boosts positive energy
- Regulates blood pressure and heartbeat
- Promotes mental alertness

Here's a step-by-step guide to chant the Om mantra correctly:

- Find a quiet place. Choose a comfortable space where you won't be disturbed

- This could be your regular meditation corner in your house

- Sit comfortably with your spine erect. You can sit cross-legged on the floor or on a chair as long as you are comfortable and your posture is upright

- Close your eyes and focus inward. This will help you concentrate on the mantra and the vibration it creates

- Start by taking a few deep breaths. Inhale slowly through your nose, hold, and then exhale slowly through your mouth. This will help you relax and prepare your body for chanting

- Begin chanting, start chanting OM, and break it down into its 3 syllables A-U-M

As you chant, feel the sound and vibrations originating from your stomach and moving up through your chest to your throat and finally your lips.

Try to synchronise the chant with your breath.

Continue chanting the mantra for as long as you feel comfortable. You can start by chanting it 10 times and gradually increase the number. As you chant, focus on the vibrations created by the mantra. Feel them resonating throughout your body, bringing a sense of peace and relaxation. I chant 108 times of deity and healing mantras (Om, Om Namah Shivaya, Lokha Samastha Sukino Bhavantu, Om Mani Padme Hum).

Once you have finished chanting, sit quietly for a few minutes with your eyes closed. Observe any thoughts or feelings that arise and let them pass without any judgement.

Guided Meditation:

Guided meditation is a type of meditation led by a teacher who explains what to do. They cue us when to open and close our eyes, how to breathe, and break down other meditation techniques because they are experts on how the mind works.

The Honest Guys' guided meditations are some of my favourites. They are expertly written and delivered in a voice that is instantly calming and relaxing. Whether you are stressed or need a bit of help going to sleep, this guided meditation can help any beginner reach a deep, blissful state of relaxation.

The guided meditations help you connect in the moment and soak in the peace and stillness surrounding you.

There is no good time to start meditation. If you want to start seeing some good results, then do it now.

Metta Meditation: The Loving-kindness Meditation

Metta meditation is a type of Buddhist meditation. 'Metta' means positive energy and kindness towards others.

The goal of metta meditation is to cultivate kindness for all beings, including yourself and:

- Family

- Friends

- Neighbours

- Acquaintances

- Difficult people in your life

- All other living creatures

Like other types of meditation, the metta practice is beneficial for mental, emotional, and physical health. It's especially useful for reducing negative emotions and resentment towards yourself and other people.

It's also mainly done to harness positive emotions. This includes feelings of

- Joy

- Trust

- Love

- Gratitude

- Happiness

- Appreciation

- Compassion

To cultivate these emotions, you silently recite phrases to yourself and others.

Metta Meditation:

- May I be Happy
- May I be Healthy
- May I be free from suffering
- May I live in peace
- May my life be blessed with ease
- **Visualise others** (family, friends, acquaintances, difficult people in your life)
- May you be happy
- May you be healthy
- May you be free from suffering
- May you live in peace
- May your life be blessed with ease
- **Benefits:** Promotes self-compassion, improves longevity, and enhances social connections

Mood Enhancer Meditation:

Close your eyes gently. Focus on your breathing.

As you inhale, take in all the goodness and as you exhale, let out all the negativities and release the tensions from your body.

- Inhale: Positivity
- Exhale: Negativity

- Inhale: Joy

- Exhale: Sorrow

- Inhale: Clarity

- Exhale: Confusion

- Inhale: Strength

- Exhale: Weakness

- Inhale: Activeness

- Exhale: Laziness

- Inhale: Calmness

- Exhale: Resentment

- Inhale: Health

- Exhale: Illness

- Inhale: Confidence

- Exhale: Doubts and Fears

- Inhale: Serenity and Tranquillity

- Exhale: Anger and Frustration

Yoga Nidra:

Yoga Nidra or yogic sleep, as it is commonly known, is a powerful meditation technique. Yoga nidra promotes deep rest and relaxation that isn't found in any other practice.

Some people crave the profound relaxation that this practice instils.

Yoga Nidra involves slowing down and chilling out.

Tips for practising yoga Nidra:

If lying down on the floor for a while wouldn't be comfortable, you can practice yoga Nidra in a recliner or even in a bed.

You don't have to start with a long session. Start with 15 minutes a day and work your way up. A night-time practice can help you sleep tight through most of the night. Quieting your mind and not doing anything is much harder than you think. So give yoga Nidra a few tries without giving up.

Step-by-step instructions:

Lie down straight on your back in a corpse pose (Shavasana). Close your eyes and relax. Take a few deep breaths in and out. Remember to take slow and relaxed breaths.

Start by gently focusing your attention on your right foot. Keep your attention there for a few seconds while relaxing your foot. Then, gently move your attention up to the right knee, right thigh, and hip. Become aware of your whole right leg.

Gently repeat this process for the left leg.

Pay attention to all parts of the body: genital area, stomach, navel region, chest.

Take your attention to the right shoulder and right arm, palms, and fingers, then repeat this on the left shoulder, arm, throat, face, and finally, the top of the head.

Take a deep breath in, observe the sensations in your body, and relax in this still state for a few minutes.

Now slowly becoming aware of your body and surroundings, turn to the right side and keep lying down for a few minutes more. Rolling over to the right side makes the breath flow through the left nostril, which helps cool the body.

Taking your own time, you may slowly sit up. Whenever you feel comfortable, slowly and gradually open your eyes.

Note: Yoga Nidra is not a conscious effort but conscious relaxation.

You don't need to physically move or touch your body parts. You only need to take your attention gently towards them with awareness and remain effortless and consciously relax the body and mind.

Yoga Nidra is a joyous and effortless way to end your yoga practice.

Benefits: cools down the body after the yoga postures, restoring normal temperature

Activates the nervous system.

Reduces chronic pain and inflammation.

Promotes deep psychological healing and emotional balance.

Fosters a sense of deep inner peace and harmony.

Mind:

The human mind is a powerful tool with so much power and potential locked inside, but the vast majority of us never learn how to unlock it. It has the power to keep us healthy and make us sick. It has the ability to block our potential or make us soar to newer possibilities beyond our wildest dreams. It literally has the power to create our reality.

I have 2 powerful examples of the 2 closest people in my life. One of my closest friend, several years ago, met with a major accident. As a yoga enthusiast, anybody dreams about being physically active and mobile. After combating several months of injury combined with infections and pus oozing out of her right hand, she showed remarkable resilience and determination towards her recovery journey from a severe hand injury. Such comebacks can be incredibly inspiring, showcasing both physical and mental strength.

The scar on her hand is still visible and so deep, revealing the nightmarish incident; she was one of the passengers in the car when a truck hit their car from behind, and the force with which her hand got caught struck between the doors of the car. It took almost several months of shuttling to doctors post-surgery. The inner turmoil she went through when the doctor suggested they may consider amputating her hand put her into a state of shock. With her strong grit and willpower, she not only recovered, she started driving, teaching yoga and cooking, and doing all her routines she thought weren't possible.

Her spirits are so high that despite her limitations, she still teaches yoga and is one of the refined teachers setting an exemplary example of 'pushing oneself beyond limits'.

Her story serves as a powerful example of perseverance and hope. Yoga often involves significant mental and physical discipline, which would have been crucial in her early stages of recovery. As a yoga teacher, her journey must have likely involved overcoming significant physical and emotional hurdles.

She has shaped so many people of all age groups into becoming yoga enthusiasts and is dedicated and strongly committed in this line of service for the past 26 years. In her 50s, she has been setting serious goals for people her age. Her story is a testament to her strength and commitment, demonstrating how she navigated the obstacles of injury and rehabilitation while continuing to inspire and support others in their yoga journeys.

The next classic example of a powerful mindset shift would be my mother's healing journey after being diagnosed with rheumatoid arthritis.

Her recovery journey was commendable and miraculous. RA is a chronic condition that affects the joints, causing pain, swelling, and potential loss of function.

Recovery involves a combination of medication, lifestyle adjustments, and emotional support. Managing RA often requires a tailored approach, including disease-modifying anti-rheumatic drugs to reduce inflammation and prevent joint damage. The first few months of her diagnosis took our family through tremendous emotional turbulence. Dealing with a chronic illness can be emotionally taxing, and having a strong support system is vital for coping.

She challenged her medical reports and decided to make complete dietary and lifestyle changes. All the people in our known circle kept advising her to get into some serious dose of medications (painkillers), but she decided to follow her instinct by opting to consult an Ayurveda doctor. For several months, she would take bitter tonics prescribed as medication. Nevertheless, her internal and external conditions never deterred her confidence.

After 8 months of medication, my mum was again advised to do her tests by the doctor. After going through the second round of tests, she consulted a leading RA specialist in Asia.

The doctor wondered why she visited him in the first place. He asked her to stretch out her hands, and after carefully examining her finger joints, he declared she was RA-free and asked her who, in the first place, made her do the tests and asked her to be on medicines. She couldn't believe any of it and left the doctor's clinic with immense faith in the power of God. Her attitude and mindset played a crucial role in her recovery. She has been a true fighter all the way through her life. Despite all the setbacks, she has always come across as a winner to me, fighting her own battles with indomitable spirit. She has been my real hero.

A positive and resilient attitude can significantly impact one's healing process and overall well-being. Her immense belief in the treatment and her mental strength in facing the challenges of RA were all instrumental in her recovery. This story highlights the powerful connection between mind and body and how a strong, hopeful mindset can complement medical and therapeutic interventions in achieving positive health outcomes.

I know a lot of people in my close circle who tend to be over thinkers.

They make severe possibilities in their mind and think about negative consequences again and again. Whenever they face an issue, they get frozen and stiff and feel like it is the end of the world. I was one of them too; nobody is perfect, and we often make big issues out of small things. So the above 2 stories give me the courage and strength to handle life, both being my real life heroes.

Spam is for you:

- If you are grumpy, feeling low, or not feeling like yourself

- If you feel your energy is at an all-time low and you lack focus and creativity

- If you are on a self-healing journey or doing deep alignment work,

- If you want to ground your energy, ease tension, reduce stress, and relax your muscles

- If you want to calm your body, ease the chatter in your mind, and get a deep, restful sleep

- If you are not someone who deeply practices wellness, then spam is certainly for you to avoid a whole slew of illnesses

The techniques I have listed in this book are relatable, usable, doable, and very valuable in everyday life.

Chapter 7

Get Out of Your Comfort Zone

To make health or lifestyle changes, you must definitely get out of your comfort zone. Health needs care and prioritising yourself. "Move out of your comfort zone" is something we keep hearing all the time.

Waking up an hour early in the morning, going to bed an hour early at night, eating healthily – all these require consistent efforts, and this can be done only if you are willing to step out of your comfort zone.

Leaving the place of comfort for the unknown is not something most of us look forward to.

However, personal growth and development often require venturing beyond the bounds of what you currently know.

Whether it's taking on a new challenge at work, signing up for a class, or making a new social connection, stepping out of your comfort zone can lead to increased confidence.

"If you want something you've never had, you must be willing to do something you've never done." - Thomas Jefferson

One of the reasons why people are lazy and want to postpone their work until tomorrow is because they are too comfortable with their lives.

Many of us are afraid of failing, and we would rather not try at all.

Getting out of your comfort zone requires confronting your fears.

Instead of saying, "I don't have time for this right now," you can always make time.

You will be in a better place to confront what is truly bothering you and holding you back.

Are you feeling stuck in a rut?

Do you find yourself doing the same activities day in and day out?

Then, it's time to step out of your comfort zone and try something new.

Small wins can make a huge difference:

Travelling to new places. Travelling is like shoving a baby bird out of the nest - you are stuck in that new place, you have to either fly or fall. Find your wings and choose to fly. Travelling will give you a great sense of freedom.

When you are too accustomed to your comfort, all you want to do is just give up and go home. But trying is always worth it.

Doing what you fear doing the most: scuba diving, cliff jumping, doing whatever scares you. Whatever it is, just do it and see where it takes you.

The price of playing it safe is huge. What's the harm if it feels good, you may ask?

Imagine turning down spectacular opportunities and things coming your way. It's something like you are essentially walking away from the treasure trove of 'what could be'.

Doing unfamiliar things potentially has some benefits:

- You could meet new people
- It keeps life exciting. There's something to look forward to
- You might learn new things
- You will become more resilient
- You will be proud of yourself for trying

For me, pushing myself out of my comfort zone was writing this book. I have been procrastinating on this for the last 3 years. Finally, I decided to give up all my fears and write. When you confine yourself to the norm, you may be blocking yourself from the blessings that God has for you.

If you don't challenge yourself or are challenged by others, how easy is it to become complacent both in thoughts and actions? So don't play it safe or choose what appears to be the easiest option.

I believe that the fear of failure is a stumbling block for many people who struggle to overcome when looking to attempt something new or make changes for the better.

There are various reasons why people fear failure:

Negative childhood experiences, the pressure put on you by family or friends, and any unresolved trauma from the past.

When you recognise that you are more than enough, you are filled with the richness of you and can tap into the joy of your life as it is.

My reflections:

- Once I stepped out of my comfort zone, I started contributing from the place of 'being more than enough'
- From that place, it was extraordinary how the world responded. I realised the opportunities came flooding to me
- I started writing my book
- Gave motivational speeches for wellness programmes
- People sought my guidance for their well-being through counselling and mentorship

- As I started helping to make a difference in people's lives, I started to feel fulfilled

- As I opened up to my own gifts and path, I started to feel a profound sense of being enough

Suggestions:

- Write a short letter to yourself validating all the good things about you, all other areas in your life where you are gifted, and how you enrich other people's lives

- How would you like your life to be one year from now? What would you like to experience differently?

- Pick one or 3 areas where you experience a sense of lack that you would like to shift

- In your journal: make a list of all things you love that give you joy. Make this list as expansive as you can. So without fear, 'step out of the comfort zone'. Experience your day with so much love, gratitude, and compassion that it becomes precious

Prompts for stepping out of your comfort zone challenge:

- Physically push yourself out of your comfort zone

- Try a new food

- Try a different mode of transportation

- Practice mindfulness and meditation

- Read a few chapters of a book that's not in your genre

- Go to a park and just watch people
- Start learning a new language that interests you
- Go to a new place in your city
- Quit coffee or tea for a day or 2
- Attend a social event alone
- Do something you have been putting off for a long time (taking that solo vacation trip)
- Volunteer
- Share your thoughts and be your authentic self during a conversation
- Take a class or attend a workshop that you always wanted to attend
- Go to a bookstore alone

COMFORT ZONE

Fear Zone: Learning Zone:

- Lack of self-confidence in dealing with challenges and mistakes
- Easily worried by what others say, feel more confident

Growth zone:

- Set new goals
- Master new skills

Chapter 8

Sugar Detox

- In today's fast-paced world, it is easy to fall into the trap of consuming sugary treats without realising the impact they can have on our bodies and minds

- From candies to soda, sugar is everywhere. Breaking free from its grasp at an early stage is important

Sugary foods create a compulsive craving, just like drugs and alcohol. Consuming sugar triggers the release of dopamine in the brain, which creates temporary pleasure and reward.

The temporary pleasures can often be very detrimental to your health. I love eating ice cream more than once or twice a week. However, I realised that eating ice cream can be so tempting that it can sometimes lead to more than moderation, and it becomes hard to break from the grips of sugar addiction. Eating too much sugar can lead to chronic health issues like diabetes, hypertension, fatty liver, and obesity.

Ever since I started writing my book, I decided to consciously and deliberately cut down on sugar. I have been trying to limit my sugar intake and savour it in moderation rather than indulging excessively.

Signs Your Body Is Addicted To Sugar:

- You feel the need to eat or snack all day long

- You are a coffee hound and crave sugary drinks

- You crave sugar during or after meals. You have intense cravings for sugar, or you crave sweets even when you are full

- You are chronically stressed out

- Hunger hits you like a brick wall

- You experience withdrawal symptoms when you don't eat sugar

- Energy slumps. You may experience an afternoon energy slump or wake up tired and sluggish

- You experience bloating because you have difficulty digesting excess refined or natural sugars

Some Tips:

- Keep a diary or journal to track your consumption

- Make healthy swaps

- Instead of reaching for sugary snacks, opt for healthy alternatives like fruits, nuts, and yoghurt with a spoon of honey

- Drink plenty of water throughout the day to stay hydrated and kerb cravings

- Read food labels and choose the food products with lower sugar content

- One bar of chocolate can often lead to another if uncontrolled. With determination and perseverance, you can control your health and overall well-being

Follow A 30-day No-sugar Challenge:

- Sweeteners: table sugar, honey, maple syrup

- Sweetened beverages:

- Soda, sweetened smoothies, sweetened coffee/tea

- Condiments with added sugar:

- Ketchup, BBQ sauce, coffee creamer

- Sweetened dairy products:

- Ice cream, chocolate milk

- Chocolate/gummy candies, etc

- No-sugar challenges recommend no-calorie sweeteners such as stevia and Splenda

Benefits Of Doing A Sugar Detox:

- Improved energy levels

- Improved oral health by reducing cavities, tooth discoloration, and bad breath

- Improved sleep

Lowering sugar intake leads to a healthy blood sugar level and serotonin in your brain, both of which contribute to good quality sleep.

A sugar detox isn't about depriving you; it's okay to have a treat occasionally, but the key is moderation and making healthy choices the norm.

Sugar detox creates a space for a healthier, vibrant, and sweeter life.

Why detoxifying your body and mind is important?

In recent years, the toxicity of our planet is undeniable. The air we breathe, the food we eat, the water we drink are all loaded with toxic chemicals. Detoxification is a process to rid your body of various toxins.

Detox helps you jump-start a more active and healthier life. There are 5 primary toxins that we regularly intake - food, water, beauty, personal care items, environment, and negative thinking. It is essential to detoxify your body from time to time to avoid unnecessary physical health issues like constant headaches, insomnia, chronic fatigue, and other lifestyle-related diseases.

Benefits of detoxifying:

- It helps in removing body toxins
- Aids in weight loss
- Energises your body
- It helps your skin glow

- Improves mental health
- Helps in getting rid of unnecessary food cravings

Natural detox processes such as eating a healthy diet, getting enough sleep and rest, exercise, and staying hydrated are some of the effective methods that I would recommend. Drinking enough water is important for general health and also for detoxification.

Just like how you go on a detox diet to flush out toxins from your body and cleanse your internal organs, it is also helpful to flush out toxins from your mind. Mental and emotional toxins often go unnoticed, but they are just as essential to tidy up given the era of digital overload we live in.

Mind clutter can lead to

- Lack of focus
- Fatigue
- Overwhelm and overcommitment
- Health issues
- Unhappiness
- Chronic stress

Sometimes you need to just get things out of your head. If you are struggling with nagging worries and unable to let go, then you need to follow a few simple and easy steps.

It's like going on a mini-vacation and rejuvenating your mind, body, and soul.

Set your highest intention.

Detach from the non-stop electronics and social demands of daily life

- Meditate

- Journal

Remove anything that doesn't align with your highest intention and biggest priorities.

Saying No to people, places, or things

(If you are not incredibly judicious with what you agree, it means you will have to say no to some of the things you truly care about)

Learning to say no with grace and diplomacy is important. In the hustle and bustle of daily life, our minds often carry the residual weight of yesterday's stress, worries, and unfinished tasks. Dedicating each morning to detoxify your mind can set a tremendous transformative tone for the day ahead.

'Self-care is a necessity'.

Who among us hasn't experienced spells of tiredness or lack of energy when we just want to get things done?

The reason why you may feel tired and depleted of energy can vary from simple lack of sleep or dealing with stress at work. So following this simple mind detox can make you feel energetic and active.

Chapter 9

Smile from Your Liver

In the English movie, *Eat Pray Love*, actress Julia Roberts visits a holy man named Ketut in Bali.

Who constantly reminds her to smile a lot and smile from her liver. "Smile even in your liver," that's what he says to her.

This is a wonderful way to ignite the feelings of joy within. Make sure you get your daily dose of laughter to keep yourself young, happy, and at peace.

Doing so has numerous benefits and is better than any drug or pill.

"Peace begins with a smile" - Mother Teresa

Trying this inner smile meditation can help release all tension from your body.

The ancient Taoists developed a meditation practice whereby you hold a smile on your face and direct that energy towards your internal organs. It is one of my favourite morning meditations. It is a wonderful healing meditation that you can do any time of the day.

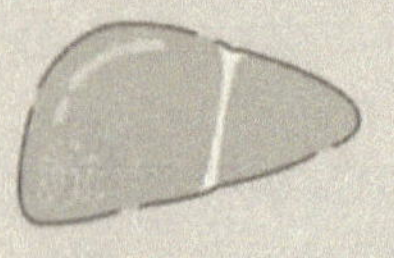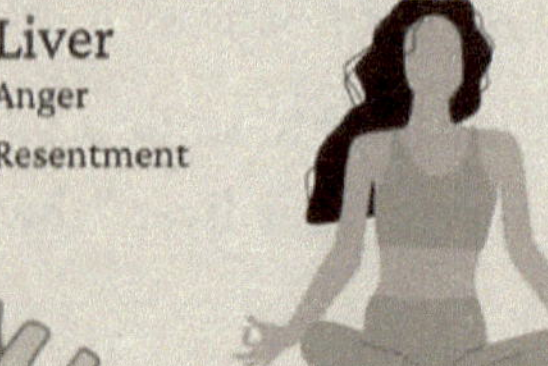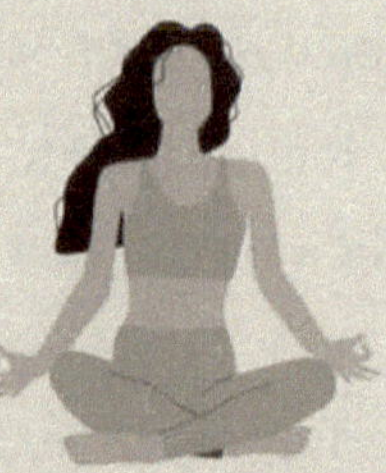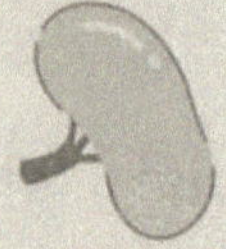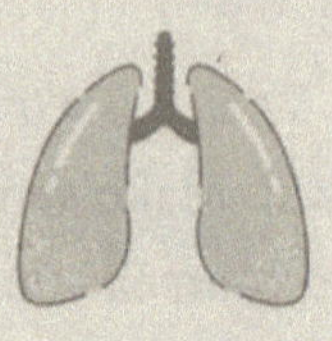

Where emotions
Are stored in the body
Liver
Anger
Resentment
Spleen
Worry
Obsessive thinking
Heart
Excitement
Shock
Kidneys
Fear
Insecurity
Lungs
Sadness
Grief

The instructions are very easy to follow:

- Sit in a comfortable position. Keep your spine as straight as possible and keep your whole body relaxed

- Take one or 2 deep breaths and fill your abdomen with air, then exhale deeply

- Rest your tongue on the roof of your mouth

- Smile gently. This isn't any broad grin, but it's a wider curve resembling more of an enigmatic smile

- Bring your energy to the space between your eyebrows and allow the smile to rest there. As you continue to smile, you will feel the energy expanding and travelling through the centre of your head

- Now, take this energy and direct it to each of your internal organs, giving special attention to any area of your body that needs healing

- Spend about 5 minutes slowly breathing the smiling energy into each organ

- Smile into your liver and release anger and resentment

- Smiling from your liver essentially means going deep within yourself to be happy inside out

- Just smile with every bit of yourself

- Smiling into your liver releases anger and resentment

- Smiling into your stomach and spleen can dissolve anxiety and worry

- Smiling into your kidneys can help you release fear and stress

- Smiling into your lungs can help relieve sadness and depression

- Smiling into your heart can fill you with joy and compassion

- To end the meditation, release your smile and your tongue from the roof of your mouth

Chapter 10

Social Media Detox

How often do you reach out to your phone as the first thing in the morning?

How often, while vacationing, is your prime focus on taking the perfect Instagram picture rather than enjoying the beauty or serenity of the moment?

Is your social media now your main outlet for leisure?

Has it become necessary for you to spend a significant amount of time on your phone before going to bed in order to fall asleep?

Do you find yourself negatively comparing yourself to others?

Does viewing other people's social media feeds make you question your own shortcomings?

Have picture likes, comments, number of followers, etc., contributed significantly to increased self-worth?

Is your online time causing you to feel more disconnected from the people around you?

Have you noticed a decrease in your ability to concentrate on tasks ahead?

Do you get headaches, feel tired, or notice increased fatigue after using social media for a prolonged period of time?

How do you feel after a social media binge?

Are you left feeling more isolated or disconnected?

Depending on the yes or no to the above questions, it might be a good idea to take a break.

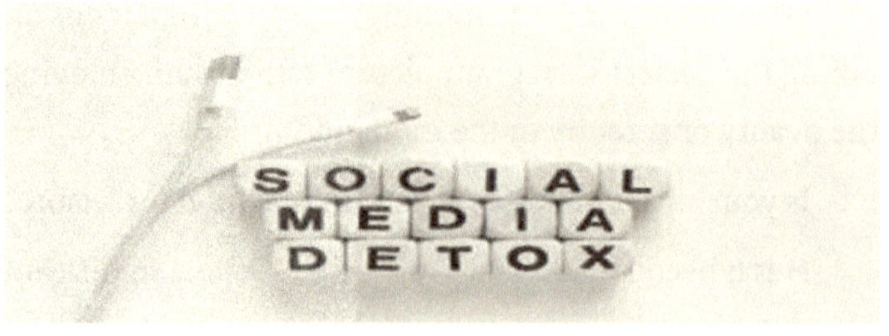

The amount of mental energy we give our phones, especially social media, could be put to much better use.

While it might be difficult initially to cut back on your usage, you might find yourself enjoying the time you spend doing something else.

Here are a few things you can try doing to ease the transition:

Start using a time tracker that monitors the amount of time you spend on social media sites.

Try to substitute social media time with face-to-face activities with family and friends who care about you. Make conscious efforts to put your phone and other devices down and spend quality time with people around you.

Try cutting down on social media at least a few times a week.

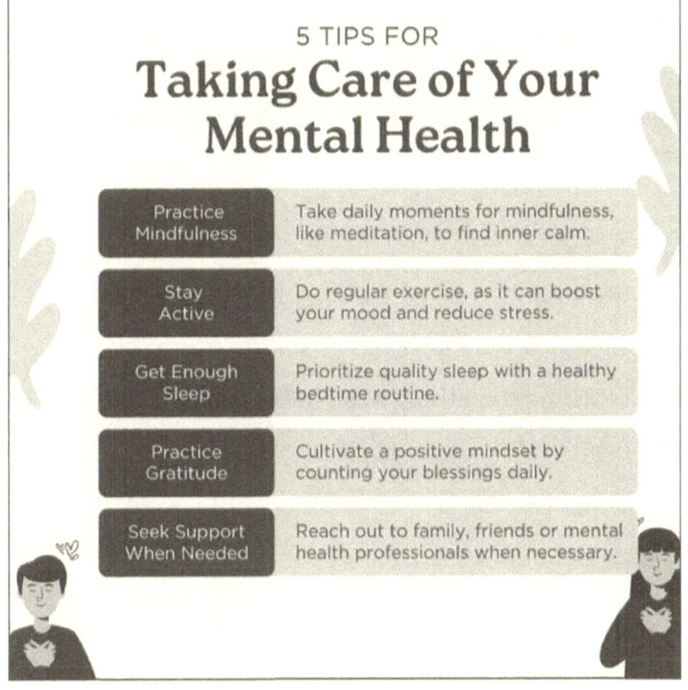

Social Detox Challenge:
- Step 1: Unsubscribe and unfollow
- Step 2: Turn off notifications

- Step 3: Stop checking your phone first thing in the morning

- Step 4: Read a book or write in a journal before going to bed

- Step 5: Have phone-free meals (strictly don't use your phone while eating food)

You may feel surprised by all the extra time during the day that would otherwise have resulted in mindless scrolling.

If possible, try to replace your social media habit with something that involves technology and makes you feel more productive.

Some suggestions I found useful were:

- Reading
- Spending time with family and friends
- Learning something new (hobby/skill/language)
- Exercising, gym, or yoga
- Volunteer
- Learn to cook
- Meditation or journaling

If you need to replace your digital habit with a more productive digital habit,

- Download Kindle on your phone and read books
- Listen to audiobooks

- Blog or write something

- Sign up for an online course

In our hyperconnected world where digital media feels inescapable, a social media detox can offer a break from endless notifications.

From scheduling a business meeting to something trivial like ordering groceries online, everything is easily accessible at the tip of our phones. A social media detox can allow you to reclaim your time and mental space.

This digital cleanse, even for a short period, can enhance and improve mood, sleep, and productivity and reduce anxiety.

A digital detox means unplugging from all electronic devices such as smartphones, tablets, and television, avoiding checking emails, text messages, and playing video games. On the contrary, a social media detox specifically targets social media platforms. Instead of disconnecting from all digital devices, you focus on eliminating social media usage. Research shows that limiting social media usage to 30 minutes per day can significantly improve mental health, sleep, and life satisfaction.

Benefits of doing a social media detox:

- Improved mental health

- Improved self-esteem

- Enhanced focus

- Better real-life connections
- Better sleep
- Increased productivity

I am not saying to cut down your time completely on social media. By limiting your social media intake, you may find yourself with renewed energy and a clearer mind. These benefits make a social media detox a worthwhile investment in your well-being.

Reducing social media consumption led to noticeable improvements in various aspects of my life. I experienced lower levels of stress and anxiety as social media amplified these feelings through a constant negative news feed.

With less time spent scrolling, I found more time for my work, book writing, and hobbies, leading to a greater sense of achievement and purpose.

Less screen time before bed, which I consciously practised at least one hour before going to bed, contributed to better and more restful sleep.

Reduced distractions from social media allowed me to be more present and attentive in daily activities.

With more time and mental space, I adopted healthier self-care practices.

Overall, you can lead a more balanced and satisfying life and allow yourself to focus on what truly matters to you.

Chapter 11

Moderation is the Key to a Healthy Living

Yes, moderation is simply the key to a healthy life. You can decide what moderation means for you, specifically. You can consider taking an inventory of your eating habits and compare them with your fitness goals. I find that it is very important to find balance in life whenever possible, whether it's between work and play, relaxation and exertion, and even abstaining and indulging. Life should be enjoyed responsibly, especially if you are hoping to find pleasure in it. You have to look out for your own health and well-being as you get older and age out of certain pleasures. What you do in your 20s or early 30s will certainly have an impact as you get older. It's good to learn about moderation from a young age.

Over the last 15 years of adulting, I have drastically improved the quality of my life using an 'all things in moderation' approach. This thought process and approach have helped me to focus on what matters most to me at any given time and let the rest sit on the back burner without feeling guilty.

My intention has always been to continue my healthier habits indefinitely while creating additional ones, and honestly, I am amazed at how much progress I make each year.

- Questions you must be asking yourself:

- Are you eating too much sugar?

- Are you dealing with too much stress?

- Not getting enough sleep?

Be honest with yourself and implement one step at a time. How did I implement moderation?

I cut sugar, a lot in fact from my diet. I never eat sweets or desserts after dinner.

I used to eat a lot of candies. I stopped buying them. I used to be an evening snacker. I realised my evening snacks were sometimes making it difficult to fall asleep. So I decided to totally cut them out. I prefer feeling less full in the evenings and rarely have any cravings at night. So when you decide to bring moderation, you don't restrict yourself from the simple pleasures of life, you just end up doing things occasionally and without giving up.

Good health is like a savings account. If you put a little something every day, it's going to help you tremendously in a time of need. Everything in moderation can create a balance for you.

Moderation can be practised by making certain alterations in life.

The first step to living in moderation is to have a well-balanced and nutritious diet.

"Don't eat until you're full" - Hara Hachi Bu

Hara Hachi Bu is a Japanese term meaning 'eat until you are 80% full'. In Japan, people use this as a way to control their eating habits. Interestingly, in Japan, people live very long and have the lowest rates of illness from heart disease, cancer, and stroke.

How does this work?

When you look at your plate, you decide how much 80% looks like. Slow down while eating and give yourself time to register how much you have eaten.

The Hara Hachi Bu method practised by the centenarian inhabitants of the Japanese island Okinawa is also a means of practising mindful eating and not being distracted by phones and television while eating.

It is about eating with full awareness and without any distractions.

In addition to the 80% formula, the other golden rules that they follow are:

- They do everything in moderation and, hence, do not obsess over calorie intake

- They eat slowly; they relish every morsel of their meal

- They focus on the food without any distractions or noise

- They choose smaller plates

- Hara hachi Bu has lots of health benefits

- Your waistline never expands. It helps avoid obesity, acid reflux, and all other gastrointestinal-related problems

Identify the most prominent things in your life that are going unchecked. The best example:

Think about everything you consumed or did yesterday. Did you eat a lot of high-fat foods, or was your diet mostly balanced?

When you use moderation, you are practising lifestyle medicine, says Dr. Brewer.

Chapter 12

Swap the Word Exercise for Movement

If you start seeing yourself as a movement person instead of an exercise person, you will think of all the small ways you can stay active throughout the day.

You will start seeing small ways you can stay active throughout the day without carving time out for a longer workout.

The less we move, the faster we age.

Each step plays a vital role in improving your bone health. However, in our everyday fast-paced lives, taking time out for physical activity can be challenging.

Affirm: I make my healthy moves every day and add years to my joints.

Inactivity has been identified as one of the key risk factors for weight gain and obesity. Exercise is often equated with noisy gyms and tedious hours logged on the treadmill. But it doesn't have to be that way. Change your perception and make it a fun part of your life.

All physical activity is beneficial and can be done as part of work, sport, and leisure (walking, cycling, wheeling) but also through dance, play, and everyday household tasks, like gardening and cleaning.

Physical activity of any type and any duration can improve health and well-being. If your nature of the job involves long hours of sitting still, then you must make it a point to move around to counter the harmful effects of sedentary behaviour. In the olden days, exercise was blended into daily life.

The nomadic lifestyle required continual hunting and gathering of food for survival.

It was quite common for people to embark on one- or two-day journeys to seek food and water. They were involved in jobs that were arduous in nature, jobs that demanded physical exertion unlike now.

So now, since everything is made to look easy and is readily available at a click of a button we have all the more responsibility to keep moving and staying fit.

Chapter 13

Miracle Mornings

MM is a concept I learnt from Hal Elrod in his book *The Miracle Morning.*

The basic concept is that you wake up an hour early and devote that time to yourself and your personal growth.

It has been life-changing for me to dedicate some time each morning to think about my goals and dreams.

Months before, I set an ambitious goal for myself to write my book, but I made very little progress towards it. The desire was strong, but the execution was nonexistent. The very thought of figuring out a structure for my writing prompted me to start waking up early.

We are all faced with the same constraints of a 24-hour day, I figured, so if others could do it, then I should be able to do it as well.

In order to write, I needed long, uninterrupted periods of time, and these are hard to come by with the distractions that crop up during the day.

That left me with one option: early morning; I began to get up at 5:30 am and write for 2 hours.

My goal was and is to write at least 1000 words each day. If I could keep up this pace, that would mean 60 days of writing that would mark 60,000 words for my book. It wasn't easy at first; some days, I didn't feel motivated enough to write. I now have over 33,000 words of my first draft written. Getting up early has made all the difference.

No noise, no email pinging, no cars honking, and therefore the morning hours are peaceful and quiet.

Tips:

Start slowly. If you wake up between 7 am and 8 am, don't immediately set the alarm for 5 am.

Waking up early is a habit that requires exercise. Every week, set a target of waking 30 minutes earlier than your usual time.

But the biggest challenge is having to go to bed early the previous night.

What does your night-time routine look like?

Are you staying up too late to get up early?

The early morning is invigorating and inspirational. It is a time for growth and reflection. If you have big dreams, it is time to actually make progress towards achieving them.

How you start your day determines the quality of your day, and how you spend your day determines the quality of your life. There's magic in the early morning.

The Miracle Morning, a productivity book by Hal Elrod, motivated me to wake up each day with more energy, focus, and motivation to tackle my goals.

The 6 practices of The Miracle Morning Elrod are abbreviated as SAVERS.

Silence:

The morning hours are best when reflected in silence. Meditation has a nearly endless list of proven health benefits.

Sitting in absolute silence for a while gives you more clarity and creativity.

My take: I committed to my meditation practice to re-centre my focus. I always enjoy 15 minutes of morning meditation.

Affirmations:

Affirmations to me are a magical tool. I use them as a tool to overcome my limiting thoughts and behaviours.

My take: I maintain a journal to exclusively practise the daily set of affirmations.

"I am an accomplished author and a successful writer. I affirm this daily."

Visualisation:

Visualisation is training your brain to see things as you would like them to be.

Elrod says, for 5 minutes, visualise your ideal life.

My take: I picture my ideal day. I visualise my affirmations coming true.

Exercise:

You don't need to run 5 miles or even go to the gym. Exercise can be as simple as doing yoga from the comfort of your home. You just need to get your body moving and get the blood and oxygen flowing to the brain.

My take: I typically do some stretches, Surya Namaskar, or a 30-minute brisk walk from my terrace. You can change the order of your practices to suit your schedule.

Reading:

Reading is one of the most transformative tools. Elrod recommends a minimum of 10 pages per day.

My take: I am an avid reader. I have around 250 books, and my passion is to build a mini library. Books have been my best companion; I fill all my free time with reading. I don't watch television frequently ever since I got into the habit of reading. I finish 2 or 3 titles at once.

Scribing:

Scribing just means writing. This could mean journaling, jotting down ideas, or making a gratitude list.

My take:

I make my gratitude list a compulsory ritual. It reminds me of all the beautiful things in life. God has been so gracious and kind in bestowing his choicest blessings upon me.

Tips:

You can essentially trick your mind by setting an intention to wake up early each morning.

At Brahma Muhurta, the mind-body connection is a powerful thing.

As soon as I wake up, I tell myself I am grateful and excited for a new day. That makes me feel far less groggy and more awake in the mornings.

These hours can bring out the best creativity in you. You might end up exploring the lesser-known sides of yourself.

Whether or not you write a gratitude list in the mornings, the mere act of focusing on the good things in your life rather than the negatives - every morning can truly change your mindset.

Sleep schedules can differ among people, with some preferring to go to bed early and others preferring to stay up late.

Night owls vs early birds:

- Sleep deficiency is associated with many health problems, such as heart disease, high blood pressure, diabetes, and depression, as well as a higher risk of accidents and injuries

- Shifting to an earlier sleep-wake pattern can open up time for many productive things

- Studies show that compared to evening exercise, morning sleep improves sleep quality in people who have trouble sleeping

- Exercising close to bedtime can have a negative impact on sleep

- Waking up early provides time to prepare a healthy breakfast

- Healthy high-protein breakfast options with low energy content have been shown to improve energy levels throughout the day

- People who don't skip their breakfast in the mornings tend to feel more alert and be in a better mood than those who skip their meal

Getting Morning Light:

Bright light exposure in the early mornings helps people wake up early and go to bed earlier. Try taking a morning walk or spending time in the sunshine early in the day to help reinforce your new sleep schedule.

All coffee lovers limit caffeine; research shows that caffeine can impair a person's sleep even if they consume it 7 hours before sleep. So avoid coffee, tea, and other sources of caffeine later in the day.

Practice healthy sleep habits to improve the quality of sleep.

Keep the bedroom dark, cool, and quiet. Remove gadgets (computer, TV, and phones) from the bedroom.

Avoid eating to the fullest capacity, alcohol, and caffeine near bedtime.

Maintain a sleep schedule consistently (going to bed and waking up around the same time)

Several successful people, such as Oprah Winfrey and Michelle Obama, are early risers.

The feeling of being in control, getting things done, being clear-minded and healthier made me happy.

People waking earlier experience a gradual shift in terms of their physical and mental health.

A daily dose of sunlight:

Sunlight is essential for life. From promoting the growth of plants and crops to keeping people warm and healthy, sunlight does it all.

Finding the right balance of sunlight can optimise the level of vitamin D. You can also get vitamin D from the diet and supplements, but sunlight is an important source.

Vitamin D is necessary for key biological processes to take place.

Benefits include:

- Improves bone health

- Reduces inflammation

- Improves the immune system

- Manages the calcium levels

Sunlight also supports better sleep and sets the circadian rhythms in the body by regulating serotonin and melatonin.

Daily, preferably a few minutes of morning sun between 7 am and 8.30 am.

- Promote a sense of well-being and improve the mood

- Relieves the pain

- Promotes relaxation

- Helps in the healing of wounds

Time spent outdoors is linked to a reduced risk of stress and blood pressure. A little dose of sunshine each day might be just what your body needs to feel happier and healthier.

These days, we are used to air-conditioned environments, whether at home or work. We sit in the freezing chill for hours together. The body gets stiff and rigid, so in order to bring a balance, you must expose yourself to these small daily routines.

Chapter 14

Sleep

Sleeping less than 7 hours can put health at risk. Getting a good night's sleep is essential for the body.

During the daytime, if you find yourself lacking energy and if you are not driven enough to work, then undoubtedly it's time to monitor your sleep patterns.

Sleep is as important as exercising and eating a balanced and nutritious diet.

Though sleep needs vary from person to person, most adults require 7-9 hours of sleep.

Sleep deprivation increases levels of ghrelin and leptin. Ghrelin is a hormone that makes us feel hungry, while leptin makes us feel full. This may be the cause of overeating.

Several studies have shown that sleep-deprived individuals have a big appetite and tend to eat more.

What's even worse?

After a few hours of sleep the previous night, you may feel unmotivated to hit the gym, go for a walk, or do any physical activity you enjoy.

Sleep deprivation can have adverse effects on our cognition, concentration, productivity, and performance.

"Sleep is critical for your metabolism, brain function, immune system, and hormone balance. Without enough sleep, your body can't heal, focus, or function at its best." - Dr. Mark Hyman

Lack of sleep is associated with many negative health effects, such as

- Risk of Heart Disease

- Depression

- Weight gain

- Inflammation

The Centers for Disease Control and Prevention highlight how much sleep you require depending on your age.

It's essential to figure out the right amount of sleep as the sleep requirements differ across different age groups.

Age group	Age	Recommended hours of sleep per day
Infant	4-12 months	12-16 hours
Toddlers	1-2 years	(including naps)
Preschool	3-5 years	11-14 hours
School-age	6-12 years	(including naps)
Teen	13-18 years	10-13 hours
Adult	18-60 years	9-12 hours
	61-64 years	8-10 hours
	65 years and older	7 or more hours
		7-9 hours
		7-8 hours

If you constantly feel under the weather and very susceptible to colds, then it certainly must be due to your sleep habits.

You must get a full night's sleep to be able to fight off illnesses.

Your body's organs work at their peak with healthy sleep.

Getting enough sleep is crucial for your physical, mental, and emotional health.

Benefits of a good night's sleep:

- Better mood and cognitive functioning
- Improved physical health
- Improved memory
- Restored energy

Chapter 15

Setting 30 Days Challenge

"Small Changes Over Time Can Lead to Big Results."

Setting any goal for a month and committing to it can be a powerful practice. Any change can feel very uncomfortable in the beginning.

We all want to lose weight. We want to get better at doing something (reading, writing, developing a skill or hobby). We all want to constantly improve but seldom work towards it.

Ideally, a 30-day challenge takes less than an hour every day to incorporate. Getting better and honing a skill comes with consistency and repetitive efforts.

For a 30-day challenge, pick any of the below:

- Run 1 mile per day
- Take a 200-word daily writing challenge
- Quit coffee/ tea
- Cut down sugar
- Read 10 pages of the book

Other challenges include:

Gratitude Challenge:

- Write down at least 5 things you are grateful for

Cut impulsive buying:

- Cut out unnecessary spending for a month

Mindfulness challenge:

- Meditation, deep breathing exercises, or simply paying attention to the present moment

Daily journaling challenge:

- Journal your thoughts, feelings, and experiences
- This can be a powerful tool for self-reflection and personal growth

Language learning challenge:

- Spend time each day learning a new language
- Use apps or enrol in an online course

Yoga challenge:

- Practice yoga every day, even if it's just for a few minutes

Creativity Challenge:

- This can be painting, drawing, or any other artistic endeavour

Money-saving challenge:

- Practice positive thinking and affirmations daily

Hydration challenge:

- Track your water intake. Notice how staying hydrated affects your energy and skin

You have so many diverse and exciting 30-day challenges to choose from. Pick one or 2 that resonate with you and embark on a month-long journey of self-growth, knowledge, and fun.

Chapter 16

Avoid Late-Night Eating:

Night-time eating has been linked with binge eating disorders and night eating syndrome.

These 2 disorders are characterised by different eating patterns and behaviours, but they tend to have the same negative effects on health.

These 2 disorders are characterised by different eating patterns and behaviours, but they tend to have the same negative effects on health.

With the advent of Swiggy/Zomato, people tend to make impulsive purchases.

People with BED typically eat large amounts of food in one sitting and feel out of control.

Meanwhile, in NES, people wake up during the night to eat. They tend to consume at least 25% of their daily calories after dinner.

In both cases, you may use food as medicine to curb emotions such as sadness, anger, or frustration.

Both conditions have been linked to obesity, depression, and troubled sleep.

Endless sleeping at night can result from a number of factors:

- Not eating enough during the day

- Eating due to boredom or stress

- Staying up late

The more frequently you perform a behaviour like eating ice cream while watching TV at night, the more likely it will become a habit in the long run.

Snacking occasionally late in the evenings or nights won't significantly impact health. With unlimited food options and crazy food deals online, it can be very hard to resist food cravings.

A lot of my friends who work in IT beat their stress by eating without control.

With changing lifestyles and the ease of getting food throughout the day, anytime binge eating is on the rise.

- Breakfast – King size

- Lunch- Queen size

- Mid-day snacks

- Dinner – light 3 hours before going to bed

That's what a day's food schedule used to look like for most of us until the online delivery.

Platforms made their way. Thanks to the growing density of food restaurants and the ease of ordering food online.

Team it with long working hours that barely allow us time to make home-cooked meals.

These days simply coming across a reel featuring a cheese-loaded pizza or burger can lure us into ordering for instant gratification; no matter what time of the day it is.

When we see people giving a must-try food review at a particular restaurant, our wish of trying the same food needs to be instantly satisfied.

The rise of eating outside can lead to the direct and judicious use of food. Regular binge eating sprees can do more harm than you realise.

Regular outdoor eating can cause a stark decrease in micronutrients, leading to acidity, constipation, dulling of the skin, hormonal imbalances, and vitamin deficiencies.

Also, eating late at night can have several impacts on health.

Weight gain: Eating late at night can lead to weight gain because your body stores the food as fat. Especially poor-quality food calories can lead to instant weight gain.

Poor sleep quality: eating late at night can tamper with the body's natural circadian rhythm, making it harder to fall asleep.

Heart disease: Eating late at night can increase the risk of a heart attack by raising the level of harmful fats in the blood.

Digestive issues:

Eating late at night can lead to indigestion and heartburn.

Blood sugar management: it can adversely affect blood sugar management.

Blood pressure: negatively impacts the blood pressure.

The best time to finish your dinner is around 7 pm, 3 hours before going to bed.

Eating mindfully and avoiding late night eating can drastically keep you healthy and avoid lot of physical ailments.

Chapter 17

Setting Realistic Goals:

Setting goals is a deeply meaningful exercise. A goal motivates us, gives us direction and a sense of purpose, and helps us feel accomplished.

You need to be more mindful and realistic when it comes to achieving goals. A lot of obstacles may come your way, such as an illness or caretaking responsibilities, that will force you to rethink what you want to achieve.

Where and how to start?

1. Deciding: Thinking of something you want to do or work towards. Ideally something you are interested in or feel excited about.

   Goals that stretch us can be motivating.

2. Write down:

   Journaling increases the chances of sticking to our goals. Describing your goals in specific terms with timescales gives more value.

   Write what you want to gain from your goal rather than focusing on what you don't want.

For example, I want to be able to fit into my old pair of jeans rather than saying, "I don't want to be overweight again."

3. Breaking down goals:

Sometimes our big goals may seem and feel unattainable. Big goals can simply feel a bit vague. Breaking down or compartmentalising can help us be more specific.

Plan your first step without procrastinating. A journey of 1000 miles starts with one step.

Even if your goal isn't to walk 1000 miles, taking that first step will help you get started.

Gradually, you will end up taking your next steps and tracking your progress.

4. Keep going and never stop.

Sometimes, working towards your goal can be frustrating, but we must persevere.

If you struggle to keep at it, take some inspiration and take a closer look around you. Take a break if necessary, but do not stop.

5. Celebrate your wins:

Last but not least, once you have reached your goal, take time to enjoy and thank those who helped you accomplish your journey.

It's indeed big to have come this far, and you need a pat on the back for that.

HURRAY!

And don't stop at that; instead, think about what your next goal or project is going to be.

Three tips for setting achievable goals:

- Make sure your goals are aligned with your values

- Make sure they are specific

- Make sure you have ample support

Chapter 18

Seven Types of Rest That Your Body Needs

Physical rest:

The first type of rest we need is physical rest, which can be passive or active. Passive physical rest includes sleeping and napping, while active physical rest means restorative activities such as yoga, stretching, and massage therapy that help improve the body's circulation and flexibility.

When every move you take feels burdensome, and your body is crying for rest, it's a sign you need physical rest.

Prioritise good sleep, power naps, gentle stretches, and breathing. Your body will feel good and thank you.

Mental rest:

Do you know someone who starts work every day with a huge cup of coffee? They're often irritable and forgetful and have a difficult time concentrating on their work. When they lie down at night, they frequently struggle to shut off their brain as conversations from the previous day fill their thoughts. Despite sleeping 7-8 hours, they wake up feeling as if they never completed their sleep. They have a mental rest deficit. Mental rest can give your mind a break from all the relentless activity.

Overthinking and overworking can lead to mental exhaustion and burnout.

Taking breaks at regular intervals and clearing your mind through meditation can work wonders.

Social rest:

Social interactions can be a complex part of our lives. Social rest involves surrounding yourself with positive and supportive people while distancing yourself from relationships that feel toxic. Social rest will allow the time and clarity to build stronger and more fulfilling relationships.

Choose your circle wisely; spend time with people who uplift you. Every interaction impacts your energy.

Carve out blocks of solitude every now and then.

Spiritual Rest:

Finding meaning and purpose beyond your daily routines is known as spiritual rest. It can be achieved through activities that allow you to travel inward and help discover a deeper you.

Spiritual rest can provide a deep sense of calm and a renewed perspective on life.

Yearning for something more meaningful and deeper?

Spiritual practices and service can resonate with your soul. Meditation, prayer, or community involvement can connect you with something greater than yourself.

Make it a top priority.

Sensory rest:

The constant noise around and non-stop online notifications can tire your senses. Dedicate an hour free from digital interruptions. We live in a world full of constant stimulation - bright lights, loud noises, screens everywhere. Sensory rest involves reducing this overload. Giving sensory rest to your body can reduce the strain on your senses and can lead to a calmer, more focused state of mind.

Listening to the morning bird sounds, embracing quietness, dimming lights, and enjoying nature are meditative and transformative experiences.

Emotional Rest:

Emotional rest means allowing yourself to feel and express your emotions in a healthy way. It's being honest about your feelings, seeking support when you need it, and stepping away from situations draining your energy. Keep cautious with your daily interactions; if you can't be your authentic self, then you will end up wasting your time and energy. You will never gain much from superficial interactions. This can lead to improved emotional intelligence and help with a great sense of inner peace.

Creative Rest:

Creative rest rejuvenates your creativity. Engaging in activities like art, nature, and music provides a lot of comfort and allows you to become more inspired. This type of rest can spark new ideas, enhance problem-solving skills, and bring unbridled joy.

Watering plants, creating a piece of art, or writing can give you a lot of solace.

Pure joy is in creating moments of awe.

Begin by introducing small moments of rest into your day. You don't need to overhaul your schedule. Even 5 minutes of quiet time can bring benefits. Pay attention to what kind of rest you need at different times. If your brain feels tired, it's probably some time for mental rest. If you are feeling lonely or disturbed, seek out the proper form of social rest. Being mindful of your needs certainly allows you to take care of your well-being most effectively. To feel recharged and revitalised, it's important to understand and practice all 7 types of rest periodically. This practice can lead to more balance, energy, satisfaction, contentment, and improved well-being.

Chapter 19

Avoiding Toxic Chemicals on the Skin

The skin is the largest breathing organ in the body. The skin is constantly breathing and absorbing everything you apply to it. Harmful chemicals such as parabens, formaldehyde, synthetic colours, fragrances, sulphates, triclosan, and propylene glycol help the product look and smell great.

Skincare with a long list of ingredients often acts as an irritant and is carcinogenic.

All the beauty products on the shelf contain thousands of toxic chemicals, and we spend a fortune to buy them.

Before you even attempt to buy a product, read the label.

Are you aware of what's going on inside these products?

Are the ingredients safe for your skin?

Sulphates are salts that are formed when sulphuric acids react with another chemical.

They act as surfactants and are generally used for lathering purposes. Sulphates can irritate your skin and eyes.

Parabens:

Parabens are preservatives used to keep skin care and makeup fresh and germ-free. They are found in a variety of products, such as soaps and body lotions.

The synthetic colours used in the products can cause skin irritations, acne breakouts, and cancer. Synthetic colours are derived from coal tar and petroleum.

Fragrance:

Fragrances are found in almost all skincare products, such as perfumes, moisturisers, shampoos, face wash, etc. Fragrances have potential cancer-causing agents.

Lead is found in lipsticks and foundations.

PEG is used as a thickening agent in skin care products like lotions and sunscreens.

It causes cancer and respiratory disorders. It can also strip off the natural oils from your skin and is extremely harmful to the skin. I have very sensitive skin, so I minimise the usage of cosmetics. Creams with SPF don't agree with my skin. They often cause a burning sensation. Before buying a product, do your own research and switch to safer ingredients for healthy skin.

Words like non-toxic and clean are basically just marketing terms.

Akin to eating healthier food, you can shift to safer personal care products as a lifelong slow process.

Our look goes deeper than our skin tone or complexion. We are not just what we are from the outside; we must be confident about ourselves from within. The concentrated chemicals or fragrances can trigger skin irritation, sensitivity, or allergies.

Symptoms include:

- Redness
- Itching
- Stinging
- Burning
- Scaling
- Roughness or dryness

Other ingredients are linked to more serious health issues such as cancer, hormone-related problems, and cardiovascular disease.

Always remember, when purchasing your skin products, you are making an investment in your body's largest organ.

Tips:

- For best results,
- Use coconut oil to moisturise your skin

- Use and try packs made of yoghurt, honey, aloe vera, and besan, mung dal powder depending on your skin type

- Using turmeric can brighten your complexion. It has anti-inflammatory and antioxidant properties

- Exfoliate your skin using natural scrubs such as oatmeal and coffee

To maintain a naturally glowing skin, keep sipping water and have a healthy diet. A diet rich in fruits, vegetables, and vegetable juices (ABC), nuts, and seeds to achieve radiant skin.

Cucumber is cooling for the skin. It replenishes and rejuvenates the dull skin. It improves complexion and reduces swelling. Grate the cucumber and add the yoghurt to it. Apply it on your face and neck.

Try orange peel; it can make your skin brighter, smoother, and glowing.

Take a few pieces of orange peel and a few teaspoons of rose water. Grind the orange peel with rose water to make a paste. Apply it all over the face and neck. Rinse it off with cold water and pat dry.

Instead of looking for your beauty solutions in cosmetics, eat fewer sugar and processed foods. Fix the gut imbalances. Exercise and sweat regularly and its curb your stress levels.

Appearing confident on the outside and feeling you are not good enough on the inside can affect your mental health.

Your physical appearance is trivial. There are other qualities that make you who you are.

Looks are not permanent; they keep changing as years roll by. You may alter your personality by changing hairstyles or dressing style. Instead of making yourself physically attractive, build your personality.

Be confident and comfortable in your own skin!

Chapter 20

Mental Health is the ultimate Wellness

"Most people don't talk about how your spirit, emotional health, or beliefs can actually help determine so much about your health. Your thoughts, feelings, your emotions, your beliefs literally communicate with every aspect of your biology every second." – Dr. Mark Hyman

Mental health is an essential aspect of overall wellness that can be overlooked.

It affects how we think, behave and feel in our daily lives. Unfortunately, mental health is still stigmatised in many parts of the world, leading many people to suffer in silence.

Poor mental health can have a significant impact on our physical health. People with poor mental health suffer from chronic physical conditions such as heart disease, diabetes, and obesity.

Stress, anxiety, and depression can weaken the immune system. Poor mental health can have a drastic impact on our ability to function in our daily lives.

Those suffering from mental health conditions such as anxiety and depression may find it difficult to focus, be productive, or maintain healthy relationships. This can lead to all sorts of difficulties in personal life.

Wellness is not just a physical pursuit. Mental health is a paramount component of a balanced life.

Chronic stress or prolonged periods of anxiety can manifest as physical ailments.

THE MIND-BODY CONNECTION IS AN INSEPARABLE DUO. Recognising this is the first step towards holistic health.

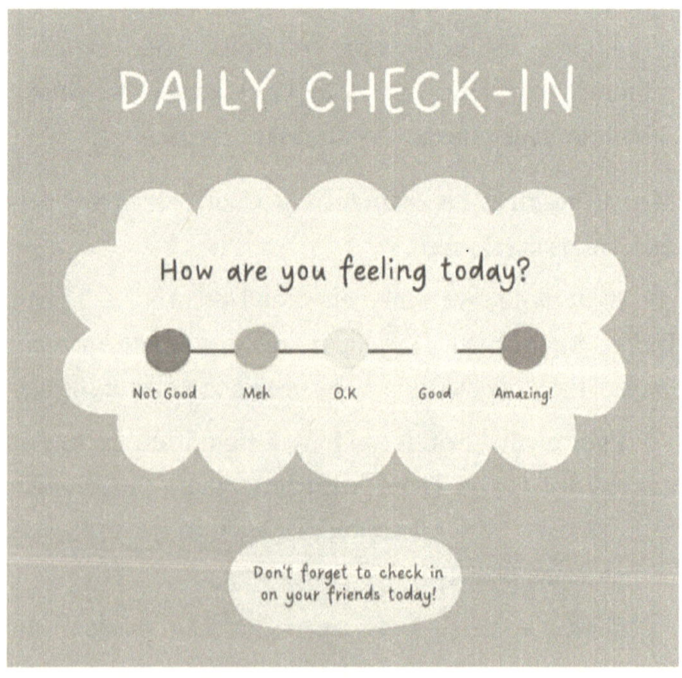

Daily check-in: How are you feeling today?

Whether you are feeling terrible, not good, okay, good, great, or amazing, this check-in is an opportunity to reflect on your well-being. You matter, and well-being is valuable.

Attitude:

The catalyst in wellness is the attitude towards life.

Challenges and even failure can impact your mental health. One must cultivate a proactive mindset emphasising resilience, optimism, and adaptability.

Nourishing the Mental Muscle:

Just as you would train your body, your mind requires care. Through mindfulness practices such as guided meditation and relaxation techniques, you must ensure your attitude remains constructive even when setbacks occur.

Nutrition Plays A Significant Role:

Food rich in omega-3 antioxidants and certain vitamins can boost our brain health, impacting our mind and mental clarity. Choosing foods that nourish the body and mind promotes a balanced and healthy lifestyle.

Seeking Support:

Surrounding yourself with loved ones, sharing challenges, and celebrating milestones together fosters positivity. Regular exercise releases endorphins, a natural mood elevator.

"I choose me, I listen to me, I honour me, I teach me, I nourish me, and I heal me."

Do a mental check-in?

Take a moment to pause and reflect on your well-being with these simple prompts.

When was the last time I went outside?

Am I being kind to myself today?

Am I letting myself rest enough?

Do I need to talk about how I am feeling?

When was the last time I took a break from my phone?

What can I do today that will make me smile?

Self-care is essential for your mental health, so make time for yourself throughout the day.

Our mental health is all about thriving and not just surviving:

Let's go from this	To this
Comparing yourself	Embracing your uniqueness
Rushing to do more	Taking intentional breaks
Burnout with work	Listening to your body
Doubting yourself	Be confident in your skills.
wanting to give up	Try again tomorrow
isolate yourself	Talk to a loved one

Talking about your problems and getting them addressed can help so much.

There's more to the age-old advice to just 'talk it out'.

Emotions can be a little harder to fix. Unless you talk it out, just speaking about your feelings out loud to another person can help.

Society has made us believe in internalising feelings rather than giving voice to them.

People often feel disturbed when they can't openly discuss the guilt or shame, which can feel so overwhelming.

If you ever come across a friend or a colleague who behaves differently, then be the reason they believe in good people.

Speaking out has powerful psychological benefits.

Talking to a trusted friend:

"I had the worst day at work" can be the start of your conversation that will help you process the stress of a hard day. With a trusted friend, you can take the liberty of venting out how you feel about your day without hesitation.

Discussing A Conflict With A Partner:

Fights are common in every relationship.

But keeping your feelings to yourself can cause a rift. Working on constructive solutions helps strengthen your relationship. Just being open about your feelings can make communication healthier as well.

Talk Therapy With A Licensed Therapist:

There's a reason people will pay money to talk through problems with a therapist. Whether you need to discuss a mental illness you are struggling with, are in couples counselling to work on your relationship or just need someone to talk to who knows how to handle stress, a good therapist can help you hash out your emotions.

Verbalising how you feel can itself be part of the solution.

When you are feeling very intense feelings such as fear, aggression, or anxiety, your amygdala is running the show.

This is the part of the brain that, among other things, handles your fight or flight response. It is the job of the amygdala and your limbic system as a whole to figure out if something is a threat, devise a response to that threat if necessary, and store the information in your memory so you can recognise the threat later.

Being open about mental health is good and allows conversations to develop naturally. After all, our stories are ours to own and share.

When you are speaking to someone about their mental health, it is important to be direct and compassionate.

You should check people's comfort level to see how they would like to discuss their experiences.

Taking care of your mind starts with what you put on your plate.

Nutrition Tips For Better Mental Health:

Prioritise your gut microbiome:

Your gut microbiome has an enormous impact on your mental health.

More than 95% of serotonin and 50% of dopamine, for example, are produced in the gut.

Tip: eat fermented foods rich in probiotics.

Add antioxidant-rich foods to your meals:

- Antioxidants help in combating stress, which is a recognised contributing factor to various mental health disorders

- Tips: blackberries, broccoli, green tea, etc

Eat oil fish:

- Oily fish is rich in omega-3 fatty acids, which influence neurotransmitters critical for mood regulation

- The best sources are found in sardines and salmon

- Check your vitamin D levels once a year

- Multiple studies have shown a link between low vitamin D and an increased risk of depression

- These days, low vitamin D has become very common. So keeping track of your vitamin D is important

Optimise your magnesium intake:

- A lot of magnesium is associated with a higher risk of depression and clinical disorders

- Over 60% of adults are estimated to be low in magnesium
- Good sources: Almonds, Spinach, brown rice, barley, and salmon
- "The greatest wealth you will experience in your life is…"
- A Healthy Body
- A peaceful mind
- And people who love you. These are the real luxuries of life

Just like how we take time to understand our body, we must take time to understand our mind. What we don't realise is the first sign of our mental suffering isn't a panic attack or emotional breakdown.

It starts with waking up exhausted after sufficient sleep, lacking motivation or purpose, frequent headaches, lack of mind-body coordination, gut issues, skin issues, irritability, low energy, feeling lost or stuck, brain fog, and fatigue. Your body speaks to you through signals. Listen to your body.

Tips to calm your mind:
- Slow deep breaths
- Practice mindfulness
- Listening to soothing music
- Spending time in nature

Just as our bodies respond to physical changes in diet and exercise, our emotional well-being is deeply influenced by our environment and relationships. When we are carrying excess emotional baggage, it can weigh us down, preventing us from thriving.

Tend to your emotional well-being like a garden. Sometimes, to help the flowers grow, we prune away the weeds. Similarly, what you allow to take up space in your life will make you bloom internally, and the results being evident that you have made healthy choices will reveal themselves externally without the need for any validation.

When we want to lose weight, we enter a calorie deficit. When we want to feel lighter emotionally, sometimes we need to be in places deficit of people, places, and things that no longer contribute to our happiness. - VEX KING

This emotional deficit might include the following:

- Spending less time with people who drain and sap your energy levels

- Stepping away from groups that are filled with drama and gossip

- Decluttering anything that no longer brings you joy or serves any purpose

- Cutting back on social media or news if it's affecting your mental health

- Saying no to things that don't align with your values or goals

- Saying goodbye to the job if it doesn't feel good

By creating this deficit, you make room for more positivity, inspiration, growth, and genuine connections. This process isn't about isolation or avoidance. It's more about being intentional with your time and energy. As you lighten your emotional load, you may feel more energised, focused, balanced, and open to newer experiences and relationships that will make you feel more authentic.

In the end, you will realise that your worth is not defined by the number of people around you but by being at peace with who you are – grounded, secure, and quietly confident in your skin.

Your worth doesn't come from seeking external validation. It comes from waking up each day knowing you are enough, whether or not others recognise it.

Rest Is Important:

- Remember, it's okay to take a break and rest. Resting is not a sign of weakness; it's a step needed for restoration and growth

- So pause, breathe, and recharge

Things that are precious:

- YOUR HEALTH - respect it, nurture it

- YOUR INNER PEACE - make it a priority

- YOUR MIND - feed it with wisdom, teach and learn new things

- YOUR TIME - use it wisely because it is the most valuable resource you have

- YOUR FREEDOM - this is a true gift; never let anyone or anything take it from you

I always feel better after stepping away from my day-to-day routines and doing something different.

I have found that even taking one day off to rest can make a world of difference.

In today's fast-paced world, people often glorify perpetual productivity. We see taking time off as counterintuitive or being lazy. However, many studies have shown that prioritising rest is not just a luxury but a necessity for maintaining overall well-being.

Rest Improves Mental Health:

- Rest isn't always sleeping, napping or just sitting on the sofa. Quality rest can mean just switching the activity you are doing with your mind (switching off the racing thoughts that make you tired all day). Constant work without breaks can lead to burnout, a state of chronic stress that affects both physical and mental state

- Taking time off allows individuals to unwind, relax, and reset their stress levels, ultimately reducing the risk of burnout

- A break can be anything from a quick stretch to a mini-vacation

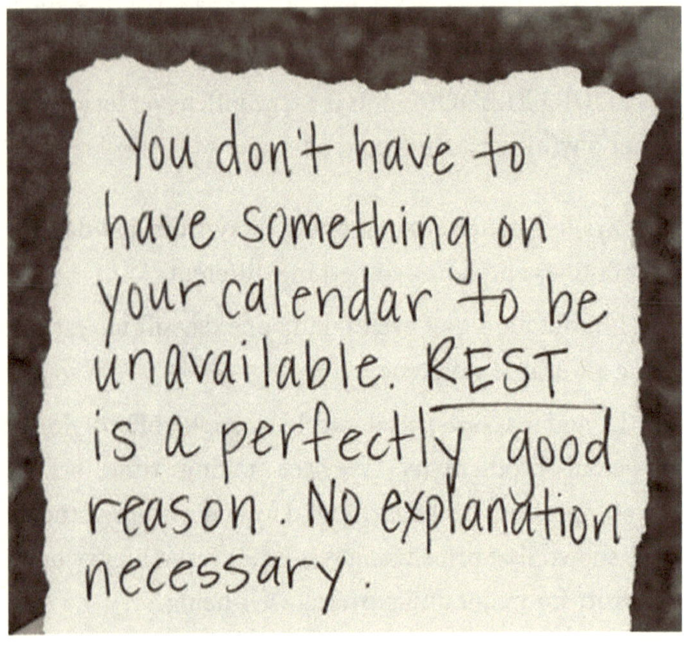

- How to rest mentally?

- Know you are worthy without work

- Schedule 'free and some me time'

- Rest = Recharge = productivity boost

- Know your place (the world goes on without you)

Burnout:

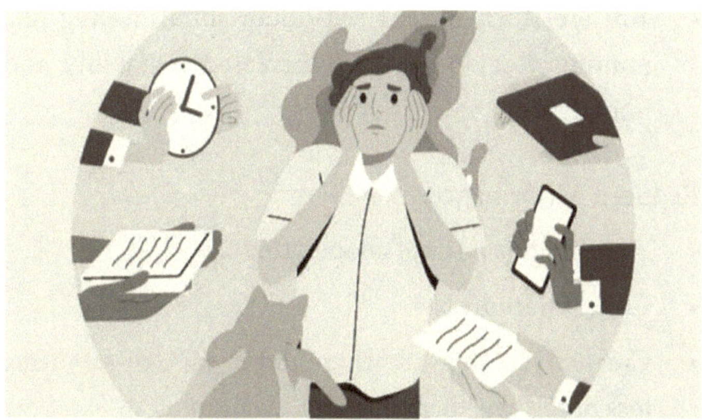

People who regularly engage in some form of moderate exercise are less burnt out than people who work out less, a study from the University of Michigan found. We need to stop glamorising overworking. The absence of sleep, exercise, time with family and friends, and relaxation isn't something to be applauded. Too many people wear their burnout as a badge of honour, and it needs to change.

Five Symptoms Of Burnout:

Exhaustion: You feel drained all the time as if you have been running empty.

Seriously, even scrolling feels like a chore, and naps just aren't cutting it.

Cynicism and detachment:

- It's like you are in your own world and can't connect with anyone. You are side-eyeing your friend's job and family

Feelings of Ineffectiveness:

- You are stuck in that self-doubt spiral, feeling like nothing you do matters. Increased irritability and impatience

Reduced performance:

- Your brain is just not cooperating

- Concentration? No

- Creativity? A big no, where did it go? Self-sabotage, loss of self-worth, and low motivation

- You are just going through the routines mundanely, and it's frustrating

Health problems:

You deal with random stuff like

Tummy aches, pounding head and sleep-related problems, insomnia and sleep-related issues, difficulty concentrating or deciding, and weakened immunity.

Overall, what a mess!

Who doesn't feel overwhelmed or stretched thin sometimes? When relentless work stress pushes you into a debilitating state, we call it burnout. Focusing on unrelenting hustle and neglecting health can cost a fortune. It can often feel insurmountable. But the sense of being overwhelmed is a signal and not a long-term sentence.

Ways to cope with burnout:

- Examine your options, set clear boundaries, make time for the things you love, practice self-compassion, talk to the people you trust, make small, immediate changes, be patient, take regular breaks, take it one step at a time, and stop comparing

Slowing Down:

I live with an autoimmune condition called Sjogren's syndrome. Fatigue is one of the most frequent symptoms, and I tend to feel tired most of the time. I make sure that I have lots of time for rest, where I am not rushing to get up or doing lots of things that don't necessarily energise me.

Doing leisurely tasks such as reading, going for a walk, or having a quiet catch-up with loved ones can be just as restful as having a sleep or nap.

So how would you figure out what resting looks like for you? I would recommend you to think about the things that bring you instant joy and the activities you can get lost in.

Intentionally slowing down for a moment and prioritising what you need without thinking too much about all other things is the first step towards your mental health.

It's in slowing down that we find healing, peace, clarity, and the joy of living. Reading slower, thinking slower, eating slower, and breathing slower. A few years ago, I came to the realisation that I was going too fast; the unsustainable pace at which I was operating made me constantly distracted and uncomfortable. The predictable result was that I had to redo tasks that I rushed through the first time. Yet, when I deliberately slowed down my approach, I completed the tasks relatively with relative ease. This led to an epiphany. Why don't I take things slower, to begin with, and be more mindful of my approach? By slowing down, I am calmer and able to focus well on the task at hand.

Self-love:
"I hope you wake up with love, love for life, love for others, and most importantly, love for yourself."

Appreciate, be kind, believe in, respect, and encourage yourself.

Society has a way of pushing us to always want more; this pressure adds layers of stress and burnout.

Don't let society push you into losing sight of your own pace and needs. Choosing less will lead to clarity, peace of mind, and a deeper sense of self-worth. When society tries pushing you with the idea of settling with more, work your way through by thinking more positively, being more grateful, being more authentic, being bold, and confident.

Self-love is the best form of love. Cue thoughts of loving the shape of your body, learning to love your quirks, and embracing all your imperfections. It's okay to remain flawed and yet love yourself. That's the first sign of deep work.

In the highlight of the social media reels, we only get to see the fun, feel-good parts. Yes, self-love should absolutely include self-care, but it must also include parenting yourself.

The worst thing about being an adult is that you need to take full control of your life; there is no one to tell you to stop scrolling through Instagram until midnight.

No one is to make you eat a bowl full of fruits and vegetables unless you are diet-conscious and care about what you eat.

You may feel irritable and not feel like doing most of your tasks. Learning to love truly is an inside job.

Self-love is re-evaluating your daily habits to determine what is good for you versus what makes you take a guilt trip.

Self-love is more than rewarding oneself with a slice of cake and a selfie.

Beyond mere pleasures, it includes deeper meanings such as:

- Recognising areas of strength and weakness
- Recognising your emotions and respecting your mental health
- Admitting your flaws

- Putting your needs first and above everything else

- Having patience and love

- Being kind to yourself even when you make mistakes

Self-love is not merely a trendy concept but a fundamental pillar of mental well-being and healthy relationships.

Loving yourself can make such a huge difference in how you experience life.

To build up feelings of love towards yourself, start treating yourself like someone you already love.

- Talk to yourself kindly

- Take care of your needs

- Eat well

- Drink plenty of water

- Get enough sleep

- Work on shifting unhelpful thought patterns, stories, and beliefs

- Give yourself permission to love your body. Your body is gorgeous and a fantastic tool for exploration

There is so much you can do while you are alive! Climb, run, eat, do all that you love, and care for your body as if it were your child.

When you don't know which step to take next, turn inward.

Nurture your spirit, heal your wounds and embrace the present moment.

Discover ways to love yourself on a deeper level:

Try practising these 7 steps for self-love:

- **Self-awareness**: understanding your thoughts, feelings, and behaviour

- **Self-expression:** being authentic to who you are in all areas of life

- **Self-care**: taking care of your body and mind

- **Self-compassion:** Be kind to yourself, especially during tough times

- **Self-respect:** Honour your worth by setting boundaries

- **Self-acceptance:** embracing who you are, including the parts you don't find perfect

Sometimes, past experiences, societal expectations, or self-judgements can create blocks on the path to self-love.

Signs Of Lack Of Self-love:

Lack of self-love can show up in different ways.

- Self-criticism

- Ignoring your own needs

- Having difficulty accepting compliments

- Neglecting self-care

The good news is that recognising these signs is the first step towards change.

Cultivating Kindness:

Kindness is choosing to do something that helps others or yourself. Kindness, or doing good, often means putting other people's needs before our own.

It could be giving up the seat on the bus to someone who may need it, offering to make a cup of tea for someone at work, holding the door for someone, or offering to carry a tray for someone whose hands are full.

Unexpected kindness is the most powerful thing. With just a few kind words, you can change someone's entire day.

The people we care about the most are often the ones we forget to be kind to. Research shows that helping others can benefit our own mental health and well-being.

Kindness has many health benefits:

- Kindness can decrease blood pressure and cortisol hormone that are directly linked to stress levels

- Kindness can dilate your blood vessels, allowing your heart to receive more oxygen

Those who practise being kind and compassionate experience clear benefits of overall well-being and happiness.

A lot more studies have shown that people who are kind tend to live longer.

It can be easy to show kindness when you post something online, but when it comes to reality, it's harder to commit to kindness in our real words and actions. With everything that is going on in the world, now is the time to create a kinder society.

Don't underestimate the power of a few kind words:

- Tell your boss he or she inspires you

- Tell your children that you love them

- Tell your friends how much you love and appreciate them for their unwavering support

- Tell your parents how much their love, care, and support mean to you

- Tell your partner how much you love and need their presence in your life

- Tell your siblings how lucky you are to have them

- Tell your colleagues how good they are to you at work

"Being kind, receiving kindness, or witnessing kindness makes us feel elevated."

The most important thing about being kind doesn't have to be about making grand gestures or spending a lot of money.

Kindness lies in the smallest acts.

Thousands of people rely on food donations to feed their families. Feeding a hungry person is more than kindness. It's a basic humanity. Giving a parcel to someone hungry on the street may seem insignificant, but it means everything to those who receive it.

Even the tiniest gesture has a ripple effect.

In the brain, we have an interconnected network of cells known as the mirror neuron system. It causes us to mirror the facial expressions, body movements, and gestures of other people.

When you smile at someone without them even realising it, their smile muscles will be stimulated. – David R. Hamilton

Face-to-face conversations allow us to form deep and meaningful relationships.

Sending kind thoughts and the right words at the right time can change someone's life.

If you know someone out there who is enduring a hard or challenging time, send them a little note to let them know you are there.

Donate to charity. Donate your books, toys, and shoes to underprivileged or disadvantaged families.

Offering a seat on the bus or train to a disabled, elderly, or pregnant person is the highest form of respect and kindness.

Apologising from your heart when you feel you have done something wrong is one of the best ways to show you are grounded. Sometimes, the people we are closest to bear the brunt of our negative emotions.

Being kind to all humans. The servers, waiters, laundromat staff, drivers, maids, and parking attendants. Look for the people behind their professions.

Be the voice for the voiceless. Being kind to the stray animals is important.

When you hear or read something good, share it. We often share the scandalous, shocking, or heartbreaking news. However, there are a lot of good things happening in the world.

We just need to draw our attention towards it. Last but not least, looking after ourselves is the key to kindness because when we feel good, we emit those positive feelings to others.

Remember, you are nothing short of a miracle!

Long-term Thinking Is The Key:
It might take 30 days to create a habit, but that can change your life for the next 30 years.

It might take one hour to complete a workout, but that will keep you in a good mood for the rest of the day.

It might take 30 minutes to complete a morning routine, but it will, in return, build momentum for the rest of the day.

It might take 3 hours to read a book or something you like, but the knowledge will remain with you for the rest of your life.

It might take you 3 months to master a new skill, but that could help you monetise in crores.

In order to build a happy and successful life, we have to not only focus on what's necessary to stay afloat for the immediate future but also continually plant the seeds of our future selves.

Working on who and what we wish to be and become in the years ahead is the road to success.

It's very common and easy to want to see short-term results to confirm that our efforts are working and paying off in real-time, but the truth is some of the most meaningful outcomes, the things we truly want to work towards in our lives and careers, take time.

It may often feel like everyone else has it figured out, which can make it feel more challenging during the times we feel like we haven't done enough to be where it takes to be in life. But the winner touching the finish line is often the one who ploughs through the uncertainty phase and is willing to persevere.

Chapter 21

Gut Health is the Key to Overall Health

Gut health is important for overall well-being because it affects many aspects of the body, including the immune system, digestion, and mental health.

Digestion:

- The gut breaks down food and absorbs nutrients. A healthy gut can improve digestion and reduce negative symptoms like bloating, gas, and diarrhoea

Immune system:

- The gut is the body's longest immune organ, containing up to 80% of its immune cells. The gut microbiome trains the immune system to recognise beneficial microbes from harmful ones

Mental health:

- Poor gut health has been linked to mental health disorders

Other health conditions include:

- Poor gut health has been linked to a range of other health conditions, including inflammatory bowel disease, allergies, irritable bowel syndrome, cancer, and endocrine disorders

Good gut health occurs when you have a good balance between the good and harmful bacteria and yeast in your digestive system. In fact, 80% of your immune system is in the gut, and the majority of the body's serotonin is there too.

This means if your gut isn't healthy, then your immune system and hormones won't function, and you will get sick.

The gut is the foundation of everything. If your gut is imbalanced and your immune system isn't working properly, your serotonin and hormones won't function either, making it more challenging to stay healthy.

Your gut is also where your body gets rid of metabolic waste and toxins. If you have an unhealthy gut, your body will struggle to rid itself of those toxins.

If this occurs, it may cause many issues such as chronic fatigue, inflammation, etc. That's why people experience symptoms such as brain fog, constipation, gas, joint pain, etc. People with good gut health have more energy.

- Poor gut health, in contrast, may lead to fatigue, stomach upset, skin conditions, and autoimmune challenges.

Many parts of modern life can affect your gut microbiome, including:

- High-stress levels

- Too little sleep

- Eating a highly processed and sugary diet

- Taking antibiotics

- This may, in turn, affect other aspects of your health

- Immune function

- Weight

- Development of diseases

Ways and methods to improve your gut health naturally:

Lower your stress levels: Chronic levels of stress are hard on your whole body, including the gut. This is mainly because your body releases certain hormones when it experiences stress. High levels of those hormones may affect your gut health.

A few ways to lower stress may include:

Getting a massage, walking, spending quality time with friends or family, laughing, spending time with a pet, diffusing essential oils, and limiting alcohol intake.

Enjoy smaller meals: eat in moderation to avoid overfilling your stomach and encourage digestion. A packed stomach may also cause reflux. Set a bedtime for your gut. Try to limit how much you eat after the evening. Your GI tract is most active in the morning and daytime.

Try to eat around the same time each day. Your GI system may do best on a schedule.

Eating slowly and mindfully:

- Be present with your food and don't multitask during the meals. Bring awareness to your food and what you eat

- What do you smell?

- What do you see?

- How does it taste?

Take a mindful pause after every bite. Chewing your food thoroughly and eating your meals more slowly may lower the chances of obesity and diabetes.

Staying hydrated:

- Drinking plenty of water may be linked to increased diversity of bacteria in the gut, as water is also important in influencing gut health

- Staying hydrated benefits your health overall and can help prevent constipation. It may also be a simple way to promote gut health

Avoiding food intolerances:

- You may have food intolerances if you have symptoms such as:

- Bloating, abdominal pain, diarrhoea, gas, nausea, fatigue, and acid reflux

If you avoid foods that contribute to the above symptoms, you may see a positive change in your digestive health.

Good foods for gut health vs. Bad foods

What eating habits determine your gut health? Proper digestion is essential for nutrient absorption, elimination of waste, and prevention of toxin formation. Include nuts, seeds, and legumes in your diet. Examples include cashews, walnuts, pumpkin seeds, black beans, and lentils. They are all excellent sources of both fibre and protein. Eat whole grains as they provide another great source of dietary fibre. Eat a variety of whole grains, including barley, brown rice, millet, oats, quinoa, and cereals. The best foods for gut health are:

- **Fibre-rich foods**: foods that are rich in fibre like fruits, vegetables, and whole grains are excellent for gut health. Fibre acts as a prebiotic and provides healing to good bacteria in the gut. It also promotes regular bowel movement

- **Fermented foods**: Foods like yoghurt, pickles, and raw cheese are fermented foods that are rich in probiotics. These foods, in particular, also help retain good bacteria in the gut

- **Ginger and turmeric**: Ginger and turmeric have been used for a long time and are known for their medicinal properties. They have anti-inflammatory and antioxidant properties that support gut health to a great extent

- **Garlic and onions**: Garlic and onions contain prebiotic fibres that are a fuel for good gut bacteria. They also have antimicrobial properties

- **Berries**: Blueberries, raspberries, and strawberries are rich in antioxidants and fibre. They also help reduce inflammation in the gut

The best food of all is curd or yoghurt; it is probiotic-rich, which positively impacts gut health. Curd contains live bacteria such as lactobacillus, which helps maintain a healthy gut microbiota. Regular consumption of curd improves digestion, nutrient absorption, and a stronger immune system.

Bad foods for gut health:

Some foods can have a negative impact on the gut.

- **Trans fats**: Trans fats are commonly found in fried items, baked goods, and processed snacks that we often love to have. These foods can easily cause inflammation, which disrupts gut health

- **Excessive alcohol**: overconsumption of alcohol irritates the digestive system, thus breaking the healthy gut bacteria

Highly processed foods:

- Chips, biscuits, beverages, additives, and preservatives can all have a very negative impact

Added sugars:

- Consumption of added sugars that are found in candies and pastries promotes the growth of harmful bacteria and yeast in the gut

For a healthy gut, following the below secrets can yield amazing results:

KICK-START YOUR DAY WITH LEMON WATER

The first thing to be consumed in the morning is a glass of full lukewarm water with honey and fresh lemon juice. It helps in cleansing the digestive tract if consumed on an empty stomach. Drinking lukewarm water vitalises you from within. This simple ritual every morning will help you kick-start your day with metabolism, aid in weight loss, and it will serve as a good antioxidant boost.

EAT FOOD THAT IS GOOD:

Eat freshly prepared food, as stale food starts losing its life force, which often leads you to feel sluggish.

Never consume leftovers or frozen foods; instead, spend some time and prepare fresh, warm food. Bananas are a good source of potassium, fibre, and magnesium that boost digestion and help prevent inflammation. Apple cider vinegar generates hydrochloric acid in the body, which helps in the easy digestion of fats and carbs present in the body.

It is helpful in reducing IBS (irritable bowel syndrome) and body weight.

EAT ONLY WHEN YOU FEEL HUNGRY:

If you eat forcefully when you are not hungry, your stomach starts feeling bloated. Only when your stomach is empty do your digestive enzymes break down the food that you consume.

Ayurveda experts recommend that you should never rush while eating.

SIP HEALTHY DRINKS:

When you are well-hydrated, it's easy for the food to pass through the digestive system.

It is recommended for you to sip warm water as it takes less time for the digestion process to happen. Water is the best substitute in comparison to all other drinks.

STEP OUT TO UNWIND:

There is a link between the mind and the gut. Spending time out in nature will improve your mental health. Inhaling fresh air outside will rejuvenate you from within. After your heavy meal, taking a gentle walk or stroll will relax your body and help in the easy flow of blood in the stomach.

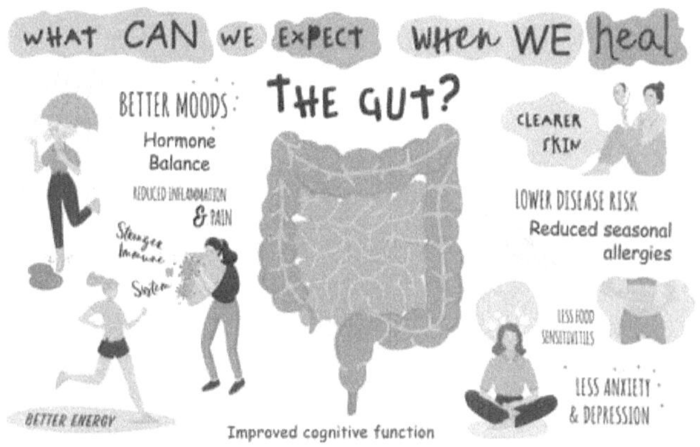

Skin signs of an unhealthy gut:

It's amazing how much the surface of your skin can reveal about what's going on underneath your gut. You may have experienced a skin allergy, rash, or skin irritation. Your skin is great at telling you when something may be off-balance internally.

Whether it's inflammation, allergies, hormones, or an imbalanced gut, your skin will respond in various ways, such as rashes and breakouts.

Signs of Unhealthy Gut
You need to know

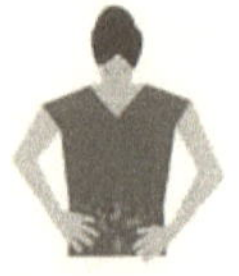

Digestive Issues

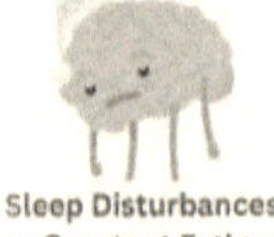

Sleep Disturbances or Constant Fatigue

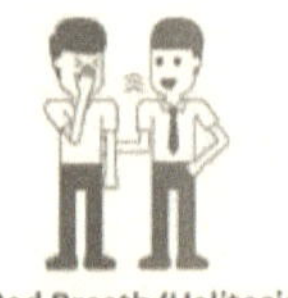

Bad Breath (Halitosis)

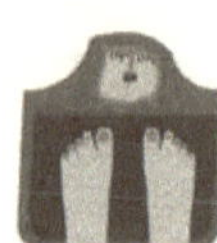

Unintentional Weight gain/ loss

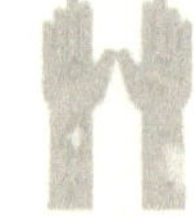

Skin Irritations

Changes in the Poop Color

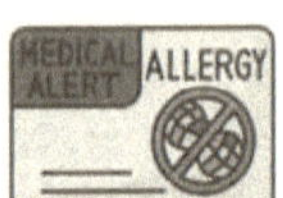

Food Intolerances

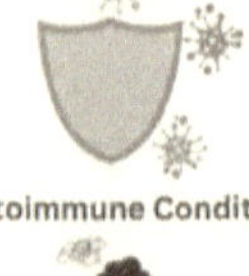

Autoimmune Conditions

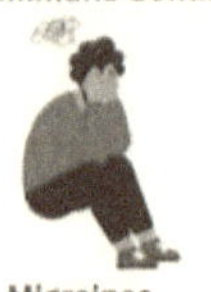

Migraines

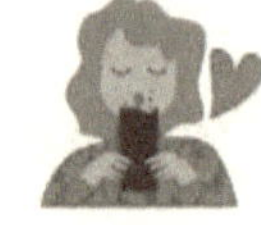

Sugar Cravings

Chapter 22

Inflammation

"It's time to realise that food is a form of healthcare." – Dr. Mark Hyman

If you fuel your body with real nutrient-dense foods, you are literally creating a healthier version of yourself every day.

Today, inflammation is a common factor in many modern diseases.

People with diets rich in refined sugar may be increasing their risk of chronic inflammation.

Inflammation resulting from lifestyle factors such as obesity, smoking, and a sedentary lifestyle can contribute to a range of diseases.

Causes of inflammation:

Poor diet, sugar, refined flour, saturated and trans fats, lack of exercise, stress, chronic infections, allergens from food and the environment, and toxins in the form of food and surroundings.

These include:

- Diabetes
- Rheumatoid arthritis
- Heart disease
- Research suggests that diet can have a significant impact on inflammation in the body

Foods to avoid:

- Sugar
- Fried foods
- Soda
- Maida
- Ultra-processed food
- Corn oil
- Sunflower oil
- Red meat
- Artificial sweeteners
- Foods to incorporate:
- Leafy greens
- Anti-inflammatory spices like turmeric and ginger
- Food rich in vitamins and minerals, such as guava and pumpkin seeds
- Limiting sugars to less than 10% of your calorie intake
- Vitamin C is a powerful antioxidant

It can seem challenging at first to eat for lower inflammation with so many inflammatory foods commercially available, but over time, small changes can turn into lasting habits.

Your most powerful medicine is on your plate. So when you make the conscious decision of what to eat and bring on your plate, you are already one step closer to good health.

Every bite you take is a chance to fuel healing, boost energy, and fight disease.

Sometimes, you may find yourself eating an unhealthy option like doughnuts for breakfast or lunch, and you might as well grab a double cheeseburger at night.

You may decide to start a healthy diet the next day. That guilt-tripping is most likely the case for most of us. Eating a few doughnuts, burgers, or pizza occasionally doesn't make you an unhealthy person.

What you do 90% of the time matters most, so give yourself the opportunity to reset frequently and do not beat yourself up for whatever has happened in the past.

We all may have some cheat meals every now and then that may not fit into someone else's definition of perfect health.

Just because you splurged in the daytime doesn't warrant you continuing to eat unhealthy throughout the day or in a row. Give the body the nutrients it needs at the next meal. What can you do to give yourself a fresh start today?

Be thankful for every meal; rejoice and eat the food on your plate.

Diet culture is all around us, telling us what to eat and what to look like. But remember to treat your body with kindness that challenges the diet culture.

When you practise body kindness, you do not have any food rules controlling your life.

Instead of counting calories, restricting how much you eat, and depriving yourself of your favourite foods, try to listen to your body cues and be mindful of your cravings.

Eating Healthy Fats Has Many Benefits:

A robust body of research has revealed the wide-ranging benefits of including healthy fats in the diet.

These include lowering the risk of developing heart disease, improving blood cholesterol levels, helping with blood sugar control, and reducing inflammation. Healthful fats have a beneficial effect on blood pressure, and they have been shown to support gut health.

Healthy fats are found in plant-based foods such as walnuts, flax seeds, chia seeds, soybeans, avocados, and olives. Fatty fish, sometimes referred to as oily fish, include tuna, mackerel, and sardines; whitefish is an excellent source of omega-3 fatty acids.

Avocados are unique in the world of fruit. Avocados are loaded with fats. Avocados are 80% fat by calories, making them even higher in fat than most animal foods.

Dark chocolate with at least 70% cocoa is also good. Extra virgin olive oil is another fatty food that is healthy. It's high in oleic acid, a fatty acid with powerful anti-inflammatory properties.

Unfortunately, many of us don't get adequate amounts of healthy fats in our diets. The right healthy fats can improve your mood, skin, hair, and nails while protecting you against type 2 diabetes, dementia, cancer, and much more.

And the higher the quality of fat you eat, the better your body will function. That is because the body uses the fat to build cell walls. You have more than trillions of cells in your body, and each of your cells needs high-quality fat.

When your body doesn't get enough fat, it gives you warning signals.

Dry and flaking skin, brittle nails, hard earwax, and achy stiff joints are all symptoms that you are not including required healthy fats.

Chapter 23

Treasure Your Energy

Your energy is a gift, and your energies are real. Invest your energy in what you want and work towards it.

Be discerning about who and what deserves your energy in life. Your energy is powerful. Don't give it away too easily to anyone. Energy includes time, words, money, contacts, and commitment.

If you end up giving it to the wrong people, you will end up wasting this precious resource and wonder why you don't have enough energy for the right people and things that matter the most.

Whenever you engage in fruitful conversations among the right people, you will notice:

- You will leave the room feeling more energised

- You will see your words and energy moving towards a solution instead of discussing problems

- You may not see a drastic outcome immediately, but you will find yourself on a worthwhile endeavour

Overall, the conversations with the right people will make it all look PURPOSEFUL.

Save your energy for those who genuinely care for it.

As a seeker searching for a simple and more meaningful life, I am still learning to be more disciplined in the things I react to and respond to.

No matter how hard you try to grow and evolve, it's always a work in progress.

What and who deserves your time, energy, and attention?

How do you stay in your light?

Let go of the uncontrollable. Take time with your life's transitions, cherish your own company, and know your triggers. Happy people work on protecting their vibe without feeling the need for people pleasing.

Hack Your Happy Hormones

Your current state of mind is determined by the levels of 4 chemicals in your brain.

D.O.S.E - DOPAMINE, OXYTOCIN, SEROTONIN, ENDORPHINS

Dopamine: THE REWARD HORMONE

Dopamine is known as the reward hormone.

It is very important for focus, concentration, and sleep. It is released whenever your brain achieves a goal. Any small goal, once achieved, feels rewarding. The more goals you achieve on a regular basis, the more neural pathways in your brain get stronger.

Ways to increase dopamine:

- Getting good sleep
- Listening to music
- Maintaining a healthy diet
- Celebrating small wins
- Doing self-care activities
- Meditation

Oxytocin: THE LOVE HORMONE

Oxytocin, the love hormone, increases empathetic feelings. Oxytocin can help us bond with loved ones and can be released through touch, music, and exercise. Oxytocin is a hormone that is produced in the hypothalamus and released into the bloodstream by the pituitary gland.

Ways to increase oxytocin:

- Playing or cuddling with a pet

- Hugging someone you love

- Giving compliments

- Doing something nice for someone

- Spending time with friends

- Holding hands with your partner and children (physical touch boosts oxytocin)

Serotonin: FOR A GOOD MOOD

Serotonin can be increased by being outside in bright daylight. It's important to remember that 90% of serotonin is formed in your gut. Serotonin plays several roles in your body, including influencing learning, memory, and happiness, as well as regulating body temperature, sleep, and hunger. Low levels of serotonin are linked with depression.

Ways to increase:

- Soaking up the sunshine

- Yoga and meditation (mindfulness increase serotonin)

- Swimming

- Practising gratitude

Endorphins: THE PAIN RELIEVER

Endorphins are your body's natural painkillers. They regulate the fight or flight response. Exercise is one of the best ways to produce endorphins in the body. As natural hormones, they can alleviate pain, lower stress, improve mood, and enhance your overall sense of well-being.

The body releases endorphins when you do pleasurable activities such as eating, exercising, etc.

Ways to increase endorphins:

- Laughter

- Running or walking

- Eating dark chocolate (a small amount can boost endorphins)

- Watching a movie

- Essential oils. Trying aromatherapy can relieve anxiety

When we understand our hormones and how they affect our body and emotions, we can give our body what it needs.

When your hormone levels are balanced, you are in a great mood and well-rested, and you will eventually feel good about yourself.

Last but not least, SMILE! Because smiling is contagious.

Smiling can help fight stress and release all 4 happy hormones.

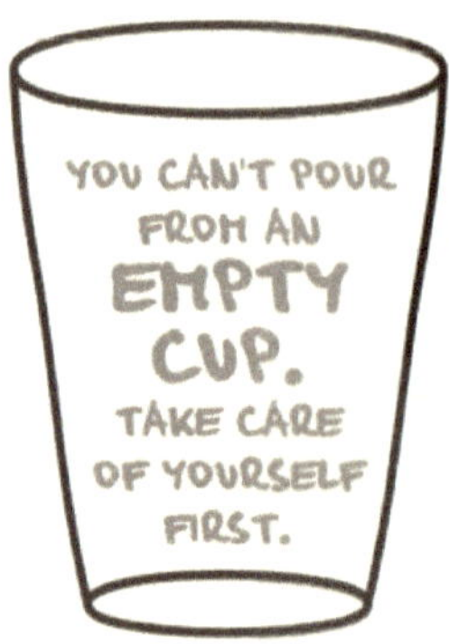

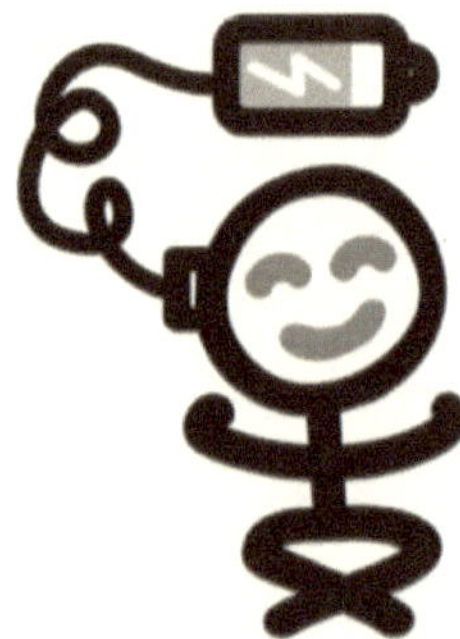

Chapter 25

Journaling

Journaling has been recognised as one of the most effective ways to reduce stress, help with depression, and deal with anxiety. Journaling is directly linked to your mental health.

It helps you open up and let go of all anxious thoughts that bother you. The best part of journaling is you can do it from anywhere. Whether from the comfort of your house or office workspace. It doesn't require a lot of time, resources, or skill.

There's more to keeping a journal than just jotting down your thoughts on paper. Research shows that daily journaling can drastically improve your health and comes with a lot of mental health benefits.

It helps you get your life on track:

- Whether you struggle with relationships, career, future, maintaining good health, or staying organised

You can use a journal to:

- Build healthy habits

- Break old patterns

- Work on your strengths and weaknesses

- Improving self-confidence

- Overcoming fears

- Practising gratitude

- Affirmations

The process of writing itself is therapeutic. Journaling can help you process and deal with both the good and the bad.

If you have been finding it difficult to live a marvellous, healthy and productive life, then journaling can be the most effective tool for transforming your life.

As a teenager or a schoolgoer, at some point, we all have had the habit of writing a diary. It was the safest space to confess our struggles, worries, and deepest fears without having the need to express it with anyone. You may have stopped doing this after reaching adulthood due to a lack of time or various other reasons.

The concept is still the same, and it is what is called journaling.

Try these simple tips to get started with journaling.

Write every day. Set aside a few minutes to write every day. Do it consistently.

Starting your day with a journal can help you start your day with clarity and focus.

Keep it simple. Carry a notebook everywhere with you, or you can even journal from your phone.

Look at your writing as a personal relaxation time: it's a time you take to destress or unwind.

Whether it's morning reflections or evening summaries, a consistent routine can help incorporate journaling into your daily life.

Choose a quiet spot without any interruptions or distractions.

Approach your journaling with an open mind. Write freely and express yourself honestly with whatever comes to your mind.

Being authentic is very important. Whether you are grappling with difficult emotions or celebrating joys, you must be true to pen down your thoughts and feelings.

Journaling comes with a lot of benefits for your mental health, emotional well-being, and balance.

- **Therapeutic**: Journaling is a form of self-therapy. It reduces symptoms of depression and anxiety during challenging times

- **Boosts immune system**: Expressive writing surely helps in boosting your immune system

- **Mindfulness**: Journaling keeps you grounded in the present moment, which is the foundation of mindfulness

Journaling Prompts:

- How are you feeling today?

- What do you need more of right now?

- What do you need less of right now?

- Who has influenced and shaped you to become better?

- What made you happiest today?

- How do you handle criticisms or negative perceptions of yourself?

- What are your biggest aspirations, and how do they align with your self-concept?

- How can you be more present in your daily life?

- How do you define success?

- What are the weaknesses that you want to work on?

- What's one life event that changed you for the better?

- Prompts to understand your emotions better:

- What happened to make me feel this way?

- Why is this bothering me so much?

- Is this emotion linked to something I don't like about myself?

- Is this emotion really true?

"We often take for granted the very things that most deserve our gratitude." - Cynthia Ozick

How often do you pause to appreciate what you have in life? Journaling brought the regular practice of being thankful for all the good things surrounding me. Through journaling, I began to appreciate things around me. As I saw more and more of the world out there, I realised all the things I had been given were not rights but privileges.

Sometimes, I write about what I have been up to that day or the previous day or important highlights of the week.

Sometimes it's more to do with how I feel. Who I want to become. More a process of self-reflection.

I fill the pages with all my random thoughts.

I use my journal to achieve my goals. I journal for self-improvement and not for others.

There's a level of serendipity that comes from flicking back through the pages of a journal. The contents may provide a smile, motivation, or demonstrate how far you have come in your healing or personal journey, sometimes triggering an idea for the next part of your life journey.

Journaling can take many forms, from bullet journals, gratitude journals, and habit trackers to tracking your mood or emotions.

Though journaling has been around for a long time, it was during the pandemic that more people got into it. The online workshops made it more accessible for people to be part of such routines.

Neuroscientists have found that writing engages various regions of the brain (self-reflection, cognition, memory, and emotional regulation).

At the end of every day, when you have recorded your thoughts and feelings, you have proof of how you have articulated your feelings.

The whole exercise of putting pen to paper activates the amygdala, the brain's emotional centre.

Journaling Helps Enhance Your Well-being In Many Ways:

- It can make you less intrusive to sensitive thoughts and anxious feelings

- Journaling allows you to reassess situations by casting a positive light

- Less anxiety

- Improved mood

- Problem-solving skills

- Kinder self-talk

- Progress towards goals

- Better sleep

- Improved self-esteem

- Mindfulness

Chapter 26

Walking

Some days, you may not feel like moving your body. 'Walking' can be done on those days. Just walking for 30 minutes can increase cardiovascular fitness, strengthen bones, reduce the body's excess fat, boost muscle power, and build stamina.

Walking can be considered one of our superpowers. Countless scientific studies have found that this simple act of moving our feet can provide a number of health benefits and help people live longer.

In the age of high-intensity cardio and weightlifting, walking is perhaps the most underrated way to get the heart pumping and muscles working.

The physical benefits of walking mainly depend on 3 factors:

- Duration

- Intensity

- Frequency

- Put simply: walk every day. Start walking slowly to warm up and gradually level up your speed

The goal should be to walk fast enough to raise your heart rate, even if it's for a short burst.

How is walking linked to longevity?

The fast walkers – around a speed of 3 miles per hour or (20-minute miles) could expect to live 15 to 20 years roughly long.

Brisk work is a cadence of 100 steps per minute to be considered a moderately intense exercise.

Walking improves fitness, cardiac health, alleviates depression and fatigue, improves mood, creates less stress on joints, reduces pain, can prevent weight gain, reduces risk for cancer, improves blood circulation, balance and coordination, and increases endurance. The list goes on and on…

Any habit that needs to be formed takes a minimum of 21 days. For the first few days, you may have to be a little hard on yourself. It may feel a bit challenging.

To maintain consistency, initially break it down into manageable chunks of time. For instance, you could split the walking routine into

- Three 10-minute walks a day or

- Two 15-minute walks a day

Tips to start walking as part of your daily routine:

Invest in a good pair of shoes.

Before taking your first stride, invest in the right pair of shoes. Your shoes should feel light on the feet and cushioned for both the sole and heel of your foot.

Wear comfortable and breathable clothing. Dry-fit clothes can help avoid the perspiration caused by sweat. Light and breathable fabrics will make your walk feel at ease.

- Warm-up: Before you start walking, warm up for a few minutes to increase the blood flow throughout your body

- Stand on one leg and gently swing the other leg back and forth 15 times, then switch legs

- Do elbow rotations clockwise and anticlockwise

- Similarly, rotate your hips clockwise and anticlockwise

- Do arm circles (10 backwards and 10 forwards)

If you want to make walking more fun, then:

Walk with one or 2 friends or in groups.

Listen to a podcast while walking.

Or listen to your favourite tunes that will make you lose the sense of time. (With 5 tracks, you would have completed 20 minutes of your walk)

Use a fitness tracker or app to set goals and keep challenging and pushing yourself.

Choose a standard time every day so that you don't skip. The key is ensuring consistency. Choose a time limit or goal that is attainable for you.

Some facts about walking:

- Walking just 10 minutes a day can improve your mood

- Daily walking can increase metabolism in women aged 35 to 50

- A daily walk can improve sleep quality and length. (Anyone getting less than 6 hours of sleep will eventually get 7-8 hours of sleep)

- Walking an hour a week can help adults improve their range of motion and mobility

- Perimenopausal women can improve bone density by taking a brisk walk for 30 minutes 3 to 4 days a week

- Walking increases your lung capacity. The morning walks or evening strolls both can have a good impact on your mood and overall functioning. This exchange of oxygen and carbon dioxide can help increase your lung capacity, thereby increasing your stamina

Simply walking 10,000 steps each day is associated with:

- Lower dementia and premature deaths

- Lower risk of type 2 diabetes and obesity

- Drastic reductions in sleep apnoea

- If walking comes with so many health benefits, why not start today?

- Instead of remaining in your seat or couch all day, get moving. Take one step at a time towards your health

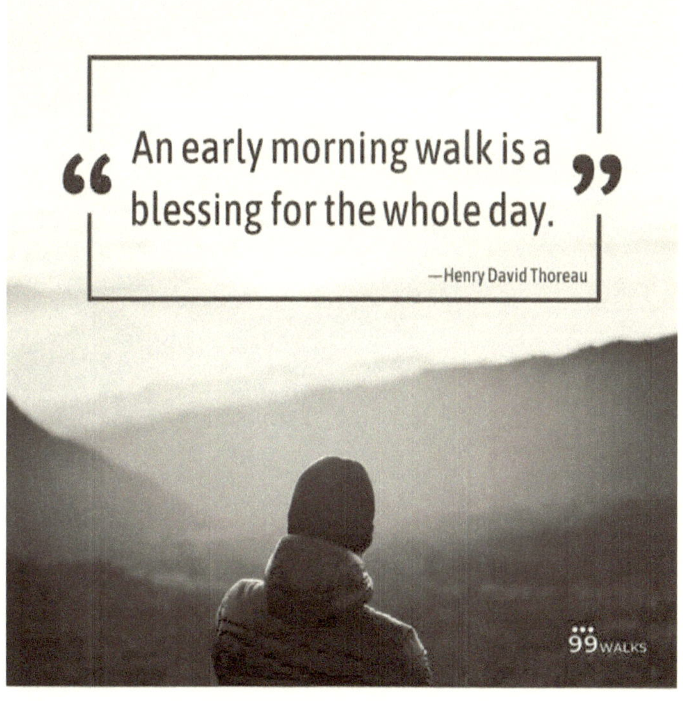

Chapter 27

Mindfulness

It's a busy world. In the rush to accomplish various tasks, you may find yourself losing connection with the present moment.

Mindfulness is the practice of purposely focusing attention on the present moment.

It's a key element in stress reduction and overall happiness. The cultivation of mindfulness is most prominent in Buddhism. The mindfulness practice is done through prayer or meditation techniques that help one stay grounded in the present moment.

By focusing on the here and now, it's likely you would get caught up in worries about the future or regrets over the past. Being mindfully present makes you savour the simple pleasures of life.

Be mindful every day in every way possible:

Eat mindfully Exercise mindfully Interact mindfully	Savour your food, engaging all your senses. Focus on your body and breath. Listen without judgement

Being present with people:

Whether family, friends, or colleagues give you their full attention whenever they talk or address something to you.

Suspend any form of judgement and listen to them intently instead of thinking of a rebuttal.

Are you present?

Is your mind full of preoccupations? It's common to find yourself disconnected when you find yourself doing the same things over and over again. Being on autopilot takes away the beauty of the present moment.

Being present with your body:

Mindful workouts can help you be more focused and strengthen the mind-body connection.

If distracting thoughts enter your mind while walking or jogging, bring the focus back to your practice, your body, and your breath.

Are you mindful or mind full?

Mindfulness takes conscious intention and regular practice.

It can be practised during daily activities like cleaning, cooking, reading, walking, etc.

People who practise mindfulness claim to experience dramatic changes in life.

They unhook from unhealthy habits and addictions.

Mindfulness at the workplace:

Create calm and focus in the workplace. The workplace is fast-paced and stressful.

Is it possible to thrive rather than flounder in the workspace environments?

Throughout the working day, employees' mindfulness is variable. They may be paying close attention in the meeting and focused on meeting their deadlines. However, later in the day, they may find themselves less mindful, staring at their computer screens, thinking about what to cook or their next plan of action.

When things get tough at work, that's when mindfulness comes into play.

Here's how taking the time to reflect on what's happening can make or break your day:

- Promotes deep focus when distraction takes over

- Gives a clear focus on solutions to problems

- Defuse emotional flare-ups in the meetings

- Empower yourself to empower others

- Helps to reduce the tendency of hasty outbreaks

Most of us spend a great deal of time sitting at our desks or in conference rooms in day-long meetings. So, having a short practice of meditation at your desk at any time of the day when you feel stressed or overwhelmed can help you refresh your attention.

Just close your eyes. Take a few deep breaths.

Inhale and exhale. Be very intentional about taking deep breaths.

Keep your eyes closed.

Have a timed session of 5 to 10 minutes. You can even do it during your lunch breaks or anytime you feel like chilling.

Do a few rounds of box breathing, as highlighted in the earlier chapter.

These simple techniques can have a profound impact on your mind and improve the quality of your work.

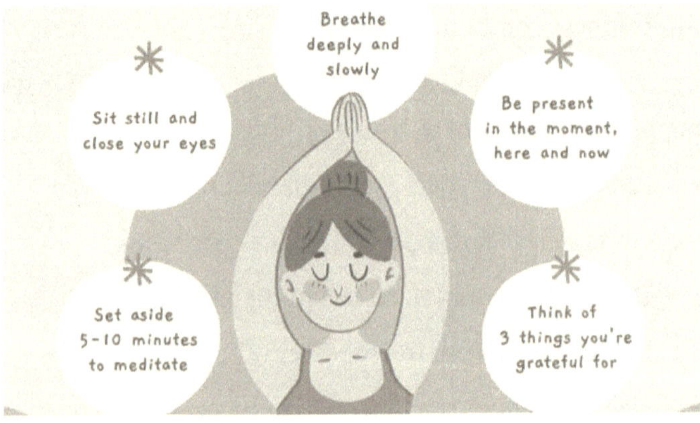

Emotional self-control is extremely important:

Emotional self-control is the ability to manage disruptive emotions and remain calm and balanced even in stressful situations.

With emotional self-control, you can manage destabilising emotions, avoid conflicts, and stay clear-headed.

However, to keep our mental health intact, we must also allow ourselves the space and time to process difficult emotions.

Mindfulness at work will help you:

- Listen more deeply

- Guide actions through clear intentions

- Behave more intentionally

- Great leaders of all times have engaged in contemplative practices

- Steve Jobs, a regular meditator, made use of mindfulness practice to challenge the operating system at Apple and enhance creative insight in planning

So many others have used mindfulness not only as a tool for increasing productivity but also for increasing situational awareness.

It's often when we want to give up that we are closest to a breakthrough.

It's often when we convince ourselves that we are no longer worth our effort, and that is actually when we are inches from getting into the hands of what we always wanted. Mindfulness will take you onto the path that's meant for you.

The more we layer our lives with distractions, expectations, and endless pursuits, the more stressed and overwhelmed we will feel.

We are often caught up in trying to achieve more, and we forget to live our lives to the fullest.

Mindfulness overall is a beautiful practice because it encourages a deep connection with the present moment. Being Mindfully present is key to a happy life.

Epilogue

Chronic disease is not a normal part of ageing - it's a result of our modern diet and lifestyle.

Small actionable steps can prevent or even reverse chronic diseases and help you age with vitality.

It's never too late to take control of your health. Improving your dietary habits and lifestyle changes can feel overwhelming in the beginning, but remember, the journey needs to start somewhere. Start with what resonates most with you and incorporate those habits regularly to bring tremendous changes into your life.

The spam highlighted in this book is for taking health seriously before it gets too late. Your body is constantly regenerating itself. Every second, millions of cells are getting replaced - skin, gut lining, even part of your brain. By tomorrow, all your cells will get brand new. So, it's never too late to start your fitness journey.

Imagine arriving at 60 stronger, fitter, healthier, smarter, wiser, and more energetic than you were in your forties. Imagine living a vibrant, highly engaged, and functional life.

We must imagine that getting older doesn't necessarily have to mean getting weaker, sicker, feebler, or more dependent.

We all know people much older, living in their 80s and 90s, who still cook, drive, dance, read, solve puzzles and thoroughly enjoy being alive. Those vibrant personalities put in effort from a young age and strived to live with optimistic spirits. When you create health, disease automatically disappears.

Why wait for a disease to strike the body? Why be susceptible to lifelong medications? You can reverse any disease through exercise and healthy eating.

Whether you exercise for 15 minutes a day or an hour, regular exercise is one of the most powerful tools you have to enhance overall health and improve your mood. Nurture yourself by doing what you love. Every now and then, remind yourself not to take life too seriously. Lighten the mood by practising the techniques highlighted in this book, laugh about things, and enjoy the fleeting moments of life. I wish all my readers a happy, content, and healthy life.

Book References

Breathe: 33 Breathing Techniques - Shanila Sattar

Wake up to the joy of you - Agapi Stassinopoulos

Pranayama techniques - AOL (Art of Living)

Kindness - Jaime Thurston

Food is your best medicine – Bieler

Tiny Buddha and calm

You Can Heal Your Life - Louise Hay

Acknowledgements

Writing this book has been such an emotional journey. I would like to thank my mother for her selfless love and gentle guidance. Thank you for placing so much trust and belief in me. Your constant support and feedback during the writing process were invaluable in giving my book its shape.

To my closest friend, guru, and confidant, for giving me your unconditional love and support and sharing your time and valuable insights with me. Thank you for being a constant reminder of the generosity of spirit that is needed for getting anything worthwhile done.

I thank all my friends and well-wishers who planted the seeds by encouraging me to write.

I thank Notion Press and its entire publishing team for turning this book into a reality. Thank you for expertly steering me through the publishing process.

I am grateful and thankful to the universe.